COSMETIC WATCH

In the same series

Stop Bingeing!

Uniform with this book

COSMETIC
WATCH

Lifting the Lid off Cosmetic Ingredients

Maurene Charlwood and
Cheryl Robertson

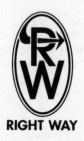

RIGHT WAY

Typeset in 11/12pt Times by Letterpart Ltd., Reigate, Surrey.

Printed and bound in Great Britain by Cox & Wyman Ltd., Reading, Berkshire.

The *Right Way* series is published by Elliot Right Way Books, Brighton Road, Lower Kingswood, Tadworth, Surrey, KT20 6TD, U.K. For information about our company and the other books we publish, visit our web site at www.right-way.co.uk

CONTENTS

CHAPTER   PAGE

Foreword   9
Introduction   11
1. Cosmetic History   15
2. The Skin   21
3. Skin Care Products   39
4. Legislation Regarding Cosmetic Products   68
5. Natural Cosmetics   77
6. Adverse Reactions to Cosmetics   81
7. Perfumes   85
8. A-Z of Common Ingredients   91
Glossary   175
Index   187

DEDICATION

To our mums, whom we still and always will miss dearly.

FOREWORD

We wrote this book for all those people who use cosmetic products on a daily basis but don't know exactly what they are applying to their skins. The labels on cosmetic products are all very nicely headed 'ingredients', but how many people understand the long list of words that follows? Most people know that *aqua* means water, and *parfum* is perfume, but what exactly are those ingredients with more than a mouthful of names? What is triethanolamine stearate, octyl methoxy-cinnamate or buxus chinensis? Mud? Egg? Chemicals? Bovine blood?

Volumes of information have been written on the subject for cosmetic scientists and boffins but we could find very little available for ordinary consumers or for beauty thera-pists, consultants, sales people and students involved in the health and beauty business.

Worldwide there are more than 400,000 known ingredients used in the manufacture of cosmetics today. (Not surprising really, since man/woman has used forms of cosmetics since cave dwelling days.) So, we could never hope to fit all the ingredients used in skin care cosmetics into a single book; it would end up extremely fat, heavy and difficult to read. We, therefore, from a cross section of cosmetic suppliers (that is, from local chemists to Harrods), selected the most commonly listed ingredients from the most commonly used skin care products, and incorporated these into our book. This A-Z chapter makes up the bulk of it. In most cases we describe briefly what the ingredients are, what they do and where they come from.

Other chapters describe some of the history of cosmetics, information about natural products, perfumes, legislation, testing and the many different types of skin care products available today. There is a detailed chapter on the skin because of this huge organ's importance. The skin reveals its owner's state of health, lifestyle and age to others. Exposure to sun and pollution, a person's nutritional balance and personal hygiene are also reflected in the skin. We felt the skin's purpose and function ought to be understood before one slaps potions willy nilly upon it.

Maurene's experiences in the cosmetics world led her to some interesting situations, which are occasionally added to the text for the fun of it.

Thanks of immense proportions go to Dr Alan J Collings and Spencer Needs for their immeasurable help on the scientific side. Thanks also to Tony Dweck, Tony Hunting, Norman Wilson, Paul Speight, Sue Holloway, Pauline Riley, Ashley Paver, Clive Bendon, Dr Bob Coombes, David Merrikin, Jeanetta Johnstone, Jill Gordon, Sandy Robertson, Penny O'Connor, Malcolm Beasley at the Natural History Museum in London, and the staff at Crawley Library. Thanks also to Zimbabwean artist Claire James, who designed the illustrations. Last but not least, thanks to Robin Ellis Mandy for his patience and caustic but beneficial criticism.

INTRODUCTION

Maurene Charlwood is an ITEC (International Examination Therapy Council) approved tutor in aromatherapy, massage, anatomy and physiology. She also lectures countrywide on skin care cosmetics and creates many formulae from her home in Guildford, Surrey, which she shares with her friendly Rhodesian ridgeback, Sula. Some of these formulae have been successfully marketed worldwide. She is a member of the Society of Cosmetic Scientists and of the Institute of Patentees and Inventors.

Maurene's interest in 'concocting things' became apparent at an early age. Her inquiring mind bombarded both parents with questions on just about everything: 'Do ants have houses?' 'Well, do they have bathrooms in these ant hill houses?' 'Do bumble bees have teeth?' and 'Do flies have bosoms?' When she was nine her father bought her a chemistry set to help channel her energy into a more orderly and scientific direction. His reward for interfering was a horrible stink of rotten eggs. It permeated the house, and 'nearly drove him to drink'. As she grew a little older she tried dissecting watches, clocks and a tape recorder (that hurt because the recorder gave her an electric shock, the first of many).

Maurene became a medical librarian, then an airhostess, and later on a mother. After producing two daughters she began to spend a bit more time at home. To keep the girls (not to mention two large dogs) out of mischief, the family spent a lot of time walking through nearby woods and fields

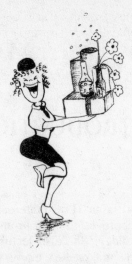

She became a medical librarian, then an air hostess . . .

where she was again overwhelmed by curiosity – this time about the flora and fauna. Curiosity developed into an absorbing hobby and soon she was administering fairly harmless herbal potions to friends and relatives who asked her advice about simple ailments including skin complaints. Developing this train of thought further, she became a qualified *aestheticienne* (comes from the French word, a specialist in beauty therapy) where her interests in herbal potions, medicine and science all combined into her present passion – ingredients of skin care cosmetics. 'My training had taught me that before commencing treatments on clients one has to buy skin care products, and having done that you have to visit cosmetic houses to learn about their ranges. I was most annoyed when the powers-that-be in these houses would not reveal every ingredient that went into each product. It seemed to me logical that I should know in detail what I was putting on other people's skin,' said Maurene. So she made her own cosmetics and perfumes, using some family formulae she inherited from her maternal grandfather, who produced various perfumes and potions in the 1920s and 1930s. From some of these formulae she researched the ingredients and began to make skin care products for a growing number of clients.

As Maurene gained knowledge in the skin care industry through personal experience and university courses, she increasingly felt the need for more information on cosmetic ingredients to be made available to health and beauty orientated students – and in fact all of us who use even one skin care cosmetic daily. There was no such information 'out there', so she set to researching and writing.

Journalist Cheryl Robertson was a cub reporter on *The Herald*, the Harare-based national daily newspaper of Zimbabwe (formerly Rhodesia) in 1978. Memories of her first assignment are deep: she had to write a piece about a bull terrier that couldn't be persuaded to stop inhaling great quantities of carbon monoxide direct from the exhaust pipe of any idling vehicle – until he passed out. Its anxious owner had to pump the dog's chest until he came to. Later she was allowed to tackle more serious subjects, including incidents in the Rhodesian terrorist/guerilla bush war. Then came an interlude in Israel, where she stayed on a kibbutz and learnt how to stab appletree-eating worms, using a lethal length of curved wire. On to Egypt and bits and pieces of Europe, and then back to Africa – to South Africa, to join the national daily newspaper, *The Star*, in Johannesburg. There she wrote general news and feature articles, and also worked in the photographic department. After four years she flew to England to go on a six-month overland trip from London to Johannesburg via 14 African countries. When the bus reached Central Africa she became captivated by the rainforests – bursting with banana and palm oil trees, plantain and cassava plants and twisted vines – and developed a passion for botanicals. She went back to Zimbabwe to become a tour guide showing visitors around the country, but then returned to journalism as an editor of various trade magazines. She later became assistant editor of one based in Croydon in the UK. The next overseas jaunt, this time with her husband and child number one, was to Malaysia. Child number two was born there, in Kuala Lumpur. The family returned to the UK and she developed her interest in the therapeutic effects of essential oils and herbs. She took an aromatherapy course with Maurene, and they felt a combination of talents was the ideal solution to the cosmetic ingredient idea. That's how this book came about, despite the occurrence of a small hiatus in research and writing when Cheryl's child number three arrived.

One of Honoré de Balzac's nineteenth century characters in *Honorine, The Interdiction*, said: 'My dear fellow, when you are interested in discovering a woman's age, look at her temples and the end of her nose. Whatever the women may accomplish with their cosmetics, they can do nothing against these incorruptible witnesses of their experiences. Each one of their years has left there its stigmata. When a woman's temples are softened, lined, withered in a certain manner; when at the end of her nose you may find those little points which resemble the imperceptible black particles which settle down in London from the chimneys in which soft coal is burned – by your leave! the lady is over thirty. She may be beautiful, she may be charming, she may be loving, she may be everything that you could wish; but she will have passed thirty, but she is reaching her maturity.'

Harsh, unfair words! While this chap may be basically correct, today there are many ways of disguising this ageing process, particularly when armed with knowledge about skin care cosmetics, the skin itself and the factors that affect it, the range of products available and the subtle differences the ingredients can make.

1

COSMETIC HISTORY

'Cosmetic' derives from the Greek word *Kosmetikos* and is defined in one dictionary as 'any preparation applied to the body, especially the face, with the intention of beautifying it'.

Cosmetic products are defined in law as substances or preparations that are applied to the body to clean, perfume, change the appearance of, protect, keep in good condition or suppress body odours. They are applied to the epidermis, hair system, nails, lips, external genital organs, teeth and the mucous membranes of the oral cavity. Products that are specifically designed to come into contact with mucous membranes include those used on the lips, in the oral cavity, to the external genital organs and in the eye area. These products do not include those that only briefly come into contact with the skin, such as shampoos or shower gels, which may unintentionally come into contact with the mucous membranes.

Why do we use cosmetics? Simply to cleanse, beautify, prevent bad odours, encourage self-esteem, or as a romantic lure, and for therapeutic effects and for stress control. We have been doing so since we first walked upright, although our ancestors used their forms of cosmetics for reasons associated with folklore, superstition, religion, fighting or hunting, and only later for medicinal purposes. The advantages of smelling sweet rather than of old goat were obvious quite early on in history – one could attract the opposite sex more successfully and become socially more acceptable.

Cave women were no doubt crafty enough to attract their men by using some sort of cosmetic, but for this we have no proof. What we do know is that about thirty thousand years ago cave men painted their skin with colours in order to scare their enemies as well as to provide camouflage when hunting. The Picts, who lived in Scotland around 1000 BC, were so-called by the Romans from the Latin *pictus*, which means 'painted'.

The earliest historical record of cosmetic use comes from around 5500 BC during the Predynastic period of Egypt. In later tombs, including that of Menes, the first Pharaoh, unguent (ointment) jars were discovered, and from remains of other periods it is evident the ointments were scented. These and perfumed oils were used by men and women as anti-wrinkle agents in the dry Egyptian heat.

Soap-like products consisting of fat boiled with ash were made in Babylon around 2800 BC, but these are generally thought to have been for washing clothes, not bodies. Personal washing soap was developed about a thousand years ago by people from Mediterranean countries using a crude basic recipe. It consisted of various animal fats (tallow or suet), and vegetable oil (maybe olive oil or rapeseed). Such a smelly product may well have been counter-productive – soap really started to evolve in the nineteenth century when industrially produced soda ash became available.

Historians have discovered that around 1500 BC women used an 'anti-wrinkle' type of masque made with mud and alum. During this era unguents were made with a selection of ingredients including honey, asses' milk, beeswax and animal fats.

The Egyptians applied henna, a plant dye, to their hair, feet and hands. They painted their eyes with a mixture of ground malachite (a mineral) and outlined their eyes with a concoction which included ground up eggs of ants. The eyebrows were painted black with lamp black or lead sulphide (galena) blended in oil.

Around 668-626 BC Assyrian unguents and kohl were popular, despite the latter being made from antimony sulphide (known to them as *stibium*), a highly poisonous compound.

Cleopatra was noted not only for her beauty and charm, but for her clever application of cosmetics as well. Creams in her day (around 69-30 BC) were extremely thick unguents comprising 90 per cent animal fat and 10 per cent balsams. Ponder for a moment on this interesting race that had acquired the skill of embalming their dead. Such a race must have been rather knowledgeable about living tissue as they were able to preserve the skin of the dead so successfully. Cleopatra was possibly the first person to discover the advantages of using AHAs (alpha-hydroxy acids i.e. natural acids) – she massaged her skin with the sediment from wine vessels.

In the Bible there are a number of references to the use of cosmetics by the Jewish people, who probably gleaned some knowledge from the Egyptians. They used cosmetics for religious and political ceremonies such as the crowning of kings and also for adornment. Infamous Jezebel painted her face and attired her hair (only to be thrown unceremoniously to starving dogs and trodden on by horses).

The early Romans were more interested in warfare than body fair. However, by the middle of the first century AD cosmetics were popular among the Romans, who developed refined cosmetics such as rouge from plants, depilatories (hair removers), hair bleaches, pumice for cleaning teeth and chalk for whitening the complexion. Anyone who has visited the city of Bath in England has seen the evidence, at the Roman spa, of the luxurious way some lived, enjoying steam baths and hot and cold plunge baths. They anointed themselves and one another with fragrant oils, whilst becoming internally well oiled with copious quantities of wine. Bathing has been performed for centuries by many civilizations not only for cleansing the body but also for the relaxing, therapeutic effects of hot water and steam, and minerals found in spas and springs.

The ancient Greeks were highly refined and this was reflected in their cosmetics. The physician Claudius Galen

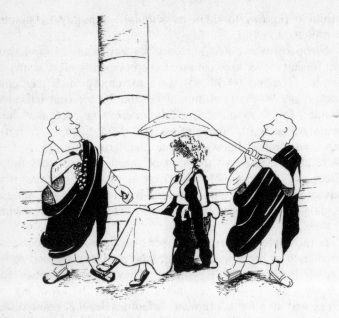

Cosmetics were popular among the Romans.

(born in 131 AD in Pergamum, Asia Minor, of Greek parents) formulated the first cold cream (an emulsion of oils, waxes and water, used to cleanse and soften the skin) which continues to bear his name in the technical term *Ceratum Galeni* (also called *Unguentum Aquae Rosae*). This second century formula which combined water, melted beeswax and cold-pressed olive oil from Greece's bountiful groves is still the basis for several creams today and is actually the forerunner of a modern moisturising cream. Sometimes rose water was added for its aroma. The slow evaporation of the water when this unguent was applied to the skin gave the product the description 'cold cream', as it left the skin feeling pleasantly cool. The Greeks also coloured their lips and cheeks and applied fucus (seaweed) to the skin.

With the eventual fall of the Roman Empire, cosmetics and other arts vanished from Europe for many years. Then cosmetics were brought to England via the knights and pilgrims returning from the Crusades with prizes from Eastern harems. When Queen Elizabeth I reigned, toilet preparations were vital to social life. Ornate boxes known as 'sweet coffers' contained these cosmetic preparations, and indeed, no *femme fatale* would have considered her boudoir complete without one.

The English Civil War halted further development in the cosmetic field. However, with the Restoration, cosmetic production and knowledge blossomed. Ladies of the Court and 'him indoors' had easy access to looking and feeling much more attractive. In France the use of cosmetics followed much the same pattern. Louis XIII used and encouraged cosmetics, but Louis XIV strongly disapproved of them. Fortunately when Napoleon Bonaparte came to power the interest in cosmetics revived, his beloved Josephine being one of those who approved of and utilised cosmetics. The industry gathered momentum in the early part of the nineteenth century, first in France and then in England. The seeds were sown then for what is now a very big industry.

Today the cosmetics industry credits its growth not only to technical advances in product manufacture and the scientific study of ingredients, but also to the fairly recent introduction of cosmetics designed specifically for men, children and people with different skin hues. The surge of interest in aromatherapy over the last ten years has added to sales of massage oils and essential oils. Although this therapy is popular now (because of the high levels of stress people encounter in today's hectic, frenetic lifestyle), versions of aromatherapy have been practised for centuries by older civilizations. While the ancient Egyptians are credited with being the true founders of aromatherapy, it was only relatively recently – in the 1920s – that the term 'aromatherapy' was coined.

Modern marketing techniques, armed with a wealth of advertising outlets, including glossy magazines full of beautiful people, newspapers, television and films, as well as impressive packaging, have led to soaring skin care cosmetic

sales worldwide and a very competitive market. The UK
cosmetics industry employs more than 20,000 people and it
earns more than £4.5 billion in sales of cosmetics every year
– a far cry from Cleopatra's day.

2

THE SKIN

Before we look at cosmetics we ought to understand the complexity of the skin. It is the body's largest organ in terms of surface area and weight; if you unwrapped an adult skin and pegged it out on the ground, *à la* big game hunters, it would cover about two square metres (22 square feet) and weigh 4 to 5 kilogrammes (10 to 11 pounds). It is called an organ because it consists of different tissues that are joined and which perform specific tasks.

The skin is the most exposed of the body's organs. It is susceptible to disease, injury and infection. The effects of sun and pollution, a person's age, state of health, lifestyle, nutrition, hormonal balance and hygiene are all reflected in the skin. Disorders or diseases are noticeable in forms such as warts, rashes or pimples. Changes in normal skin colour indicate homeostatic imbalances in the body (for example, a bluish or cyanotic skin hue indicates the blood is not gathering enough oxygen from the lungs); blushing or sweating are also noticed via the skin.

Being part of the body it is vital that it and all internal functions are working correctly. It is equally important for cosmetic users to know what they are applying directly onto the skin. If users slap potions on without thinking and do not question what they consist of, the end result may not be quite what was desired. Much research goes into developing formulae for skin care products which suit every skin type, of which there are four main categories, namely normal, oily, dry and combination.

FUNCTIONS OF THE SKIN

Protection. The skin protects underlying tissues from harmful compounds, ultra violet radiation, water loss and external mechanical abrasions.

Sensation. Within the skin are thousands of nerve receptors or endings which detect stimuli relating to pain, pressure, touch and temperature.

Temperature regulation. When the outside temperature is high, the body produces sweat which evaporates from the skin's surface, so keeping the body temperature down. When the temperature outside is low, the body's production of sweat decreases to help conserve heat. These functions in turn regulate moisture loss.

Excretion. Heat, water, bodily salts and waste materials (this includes alcoholic aftermaths) – the result of metabolic activities – are lost through sweating via the sweat glands (sudoriferous glands), of which there are three to four million in a body. Oil glands (sebaceous glands) are connected to hair follicles and secrete an oily substance called sebum.

Immunity. The Langerhans cells, found in the epidermis of the skin, are immune protectors, designed to ward off threats to the immune system. They team up with white blood cells, and are easily damaged by UV radiation.

Reservoir of blood. There is within the skin a vast network of blood vessels that carry about 10 per cent of the body's total blood flow.

Synthesis of Vitamin D. Small amounts of ultra violet radiation on the skin enable Vitamin D to be synthesised in the skin.

STRUCTURE OF THE SKIN

The skin is made up of two main parts: the outer part called the **epidermis**, and the deeper **dermis**.

The Epidermis

'Epi' comes from the Greek meaning 'over'. 'Dermis' is derived from the Greek word for 'skin'. The epidermis is the most superficial layer. It is very thin, varying from around 1.6mm on the soles of the feet to 0.04mm on the eyelids. It is of great interest to cosmetic scientists as it reflects conditions such as sensitivity, ageing, pigmentation, photo-damage and dehydration. Only in completely understanding these processes can the appropriate products be formulated.

The epidermis contains four main types of cells: keratinocytes, melanocytes, Langerhans cells and Merkel cells. It is made up of five main layers – from the most superficial to the deepest they are known as the **stratum corneum** (or horny layer), **stratum lucidum**, **stratum granulosum**, **stratum spinosum** and **stratum basale**. In a nutshell, cells develop at the bottom layer (i.e. stratum basale) and gradually migrate upwards to the surface where they finally become keratinised and slough off. The entire process from 'birth' to 'death' takes between two and four weeks. So when you look into a mirror, what you see is the uppermost layer, composed of dead cells which are constantly being shed. Were it not for the continual shedding of those dead cells just imagine what you would look like. The next (or first) time you clean the top of the wardrobe have a look at the pile of dust. Much of it will be discarded skin.

The purpose of skin care cosmetics is to put a protective layer on the surface of the skin and keep it moisturised. It is particularly important for cosmetics manufactured for ageing skins to contain elements that help the epidermis retain its natural moisture.

The Dermis

Beneath the epidermis lies the much thicker, second principal part of the skin, the dermis. This rests on connective tissue comprising a fibrous protein called collagen and elastin fibres. Connective tissue is the most widely spread tissue in the body which binds together and supports other body tissue as well as helping to protect and insulate internal organs. The dermis has two principal functions: it nourishes the epidermis, via a network of blood vessels, and it forms a support frame of collagen and elastin protein fibres that give the skin its elasticity. The scale of elasticity depends on the water content of the dermis and other skin layers, and so a dermis that functions correctly is a vital key to maintaining a youthful appearance and healthy-looking skin. Aged skin is noticeable by its poor elasticity and sagging, with wrinkles mainly caused by dryness as the oil glands decrease their oil production.

The dermis is very thick (1-2mm) on the palms of the hands and soles of the feet; while extremely thin around the lips, eyes, scrotum and penis (around 0.5mm). It is generally thicker on the dorsal rather than the ventral parts of the body. Also in this layer are blood vessels, nerves, nerve endings, lymph canals, hair follicles, sweat glands, oil glands and small muscles.

The main cells in the dermis are fibroblasts, macrophages and adipocytes. It consists of three main layers – from the most superficial to the deepest they are the **papillary layer**, the **reticular layer** and the **subcutaneous layer** (also called the hypodermis or superficial fascia).

The Anatomy of Skin
In one square centimetre of skin there are about 3 million cells, 9 hairs, 13 oil glands, 2.75 metres of nerves, 100 sweat glands, 1 metre of blood vessels and thousands of sensory cells, so you can see why it is so important to keep your skin healthy.

The epidermis is the outer layer containing nerves but not blood vessels. The dermis holds most of the skin functions in connective tissue. The **hair shaft** lies in a **hair follicle**, attached to which are **erector pilli muscles** that contract in response to cold or fear. **Oil (sebaceous) glands** are connected to hair follicles, and secrete an oily substance called sebum. There are also **sweat (sudoriferous) glands** that empty waste products including salts, urea and water onto the skin's surface via the **sweat duct**. **Sensory nerve endings** are sensitive to touch, temperature and pain. **Blood vessels** help dissipate heat from the body. The dermis holds vast numbers of blood vessels, which carry 8-10 per cent of the total blood flow in an adult when at rest. One of the body's main fat deposits is known as **adipose tissue** and lies beneath the skin.

HOW TO LOOK AFTER THE SKIN

The aim of a skin care moisturising product is to prevent the stratum corneum from dehydrating. It does this by adding an occlusive oily layer onto the surface of the stratum corneum, so slowing water permeation through the skin. Another way of increasing its water content is to add hygroscopic materials to the product, and these bind and retain water in the stratum corneum. Ingredients in a skin care product should not penetrate beyond the epidermal junction into the dermis. An ingredient's penetration rate of the epidermal layers can depend on the thickness and general state of health of the stratum corneum, as well as the molecular size of the ingredient, the evaporation ability of the ingredient, whether the skin hydration is successful and whether an ingredient blends successfully with others used in the product – if not, it tends to remain on the surface. A thin and therefore dry stratum corneum, with an uneven cell arrangement and consequent barrier loss, allows in substances more easily than normal skin. Ingredients can also move easily through a skin that is over-moist because the protective barrier has been softened. This barrier can be affected by other factors including the application of strong acne products, the presence of alpha-hydroxy acids, skin diseases and illness such as diabetes, all of which may increase product penetration. Penetration of ingredients also varies on different parts of the body – the face and scalp allow more rapid absorption than other parts. A well-balanced skin is vital – again, the aim of skin care cosmetics.

An ingredient which is said to benefit the stratum corneum by regulating the moisture content is referred to as an NMF (**Natural Moisturising Factor**). This comprises a combination of amino acids, derivatives of amino acids and minerals. Here are some of them: urea, uric acid, ammonia, lactate, citrate, creatinine, glucosanine, pyrrolidone carboxylic acid, potassium phosphate, sugar, organic acids and peptides.

The optimum moisture content of the epidermis is 15 per cent, while that of the dermis is 85 per cent, so the moisture balance of the skin is very important. To have a healthy skin, the dead surface must be kept moist (therefore soft and supple) and the live cells in the main layer beneath the surface must be kept healthy. The one factor common to both necessities is our old friend **water**. Drinking lots of water each day may result in hogging the loo but it will improve the skin as well as flush through a great deal of waste products. Blood, which mainly consists of water, brings oxygen and nourishment to cells via the system of capillaries and intercellular fluid in the dermis and in the epidermis, where the cells are gradually changing from their original composition – that of being healthy and succulent – to eventually dying to form the horny layer. The function of water is to keep the dead and dying cells soft; thus the skin will be smooth and soft. The skin of people living in countries with high humidity (greater than 80 per cent relative humidity) is well hydrated, so much so that often a moisturiser is never needed. The skin can absorb water well: if one languishes in a bath for a long time the result is (temporary) wrinkly prune-like skin on the hands and feet – this is due to hydration of the horny layers and their subsequent elongation, hence the wrinkles.

A moisturising product should either add water to the outer layer or help to keep it there. For example, apart from being rather too occlusive, petroleum jelly or petrolatum (i.e. Vaseline) is an excellent moisture retainer but left on too long or used solely will occlude the skin and can then cause blocked pores. Petrolatum is, however, used successfully in combination with other ingredients in many moisturising products.

As skin types are varied, ideally people ought to consult a well-qualified adviser if they want to find out how to look after their skin. An aestheticienne who has a good grounding in dermatology is best. Beware cosmetic sales people with slight knowledge who simply want to sell their company products.

A Few Basic Guidelines
*   Eliminate stress as much as possible.
*   Avoid or protect against the sun.
*   Ensure a healthy diet.
*   Drink plenty of water every day.
*   Exercise daily (outside if possible).
*   Avoid, whenever possible, environmental hazards such as pollution.
*   Use the correct cosmetic regime to suit your own requirements.
*   Be happy!

OTHER FACTORS AFFECTING SKIN
The pH Balance
On the skin's surface is a natural film called the **acid mantle**, formed by a mixture of secretions from the oil and sweat glands in the dermis. This mantle, with a mildly acidic average pH of between 5.5 and 6.5, helps prevent evaporation and protects the skin from certain bacteria that prefer an alkaline environment. The skin of younger people is able to return to its normal state quickly if cleaned daily with alkaline products, but from the age of 40 onwards the skin takes up to eight hours to regain its natural pH after being assailed by alkaline products. All soap is alkaline and as such is in opposition to the skin's natural chemistry. The skin is in a healthy condition when it is on the slightly acidic side.

Measuring an aqueous solution's acidity or alkalinity is worked out on the pH scale (pH = potential of hydrogen in a water substance) which numbers from 0 to 14. In the centre of the scale is 7 which is described as neutral. (Pure distilled water has a pH of 7.) From 7 downwards on the scale until 0 each step down becomes more acidic. From 7 upward to 14, each step up becomes more alkaline. Healthy skin has an average pH of 5.5, so when you see 'pH balanced' on a product this should mean that the product complies with the skin's acidic requirement.

The pH Scale		
	pH	
	0	**a very weak hydrochloric acid solution (0.0)**
	1	
	2	
increasingly	**3**	**wine (3.5)**
acidic	**4**	
solution	**5**	**black coffee (5.0)**
	6	**milk (6.6)**
NEUTRAL	**7**	**distilled water (7.0)** **blood (7.4)**
	8	
	9	**toothpaste (9.9)**
increasingly	**10**	**most soaps (10)** **milk of magnesia (10.5)**
alkaline	**11**	
	12	
	13	
	14	**a very weak sodium hydroxide solution (14.0)**

This logarithmic scale is based on the concentration of $H+$ (hydrogen ions) in a solution expressed in chemical units called moles per litre. Each number is ten times the acidity or alkalinity of the previous one. A pH of 7 means that a solution contains equal numbers of hydrogen and hydroxyl ions, and hence is neutral.

Skin Types (relating to cosmetics)
Defining your correct skin type is essential to finding the
right products. As mentioned earlier, there are four main
classifications of skin types.

Normal skin is smooth and firm due to healthy connective
tissue and good muscle tone. There are no visible lines or
large pores and, due to the correct balance of moisture and
sebum, the skin is of a matt appearance. Blood circulation is
good. Collagen, elastin and the ground substance (i.e. the
matrix of connective tissue in which various cells and fibres
are embedded) in the dermis is at a premium.

Oily skin is caused by over secretion of sebum by the
sebaceous glands lying in the dermis. Most susceptible parts
are the forehead, nose and chin, which become shiny. Pores
tend to be enlarged. Blemishes and skin disorders such as
acne vulgaris may result if the oiliness worsens. Oily skin is
sluggish looking, with an unhealthy hue.

Dry skin is taut looking, with thin epidermal layers. It is
prone to lines and wrinkles, particularly noticeable around
the eyes, mouth and on the neck. The appearance of the
skin is transparent, with the addition sometimes of flaky
skin and broken capillaries. It is dehydrated, with an
incorrect balance between moisture and sebum. Muscle tone
is also lacking. Collagen, elastin and ground substance are
lessened.

Combination skin has dry and oily areas that follow a
T-shaped pattern, starting at the forehead, running down the
nose and over the chin. The 'T-zone' area is susceptible to
over-production of sebum. On all other areas the skin could
be normal or dry, varying from person to person.

In addition, there is **couperose** skin, which is character-
ised by the face being permanently red, unfortunately
suggesting a 'boozy' look. Tiny red lines (dilated blood
vessels) appear particularly on the cheeks, nose and sometimes on the chin. **Sensitive** skin is taut, feels and looks
chaffed and is noticeably reddened. It is also subject to
over-heating. **Pigmentation** of skin appears when melanin
is unevenly distributed.

Things that Thrive on the Skin

Wherever we go we are not alone. Our skin harbours a whole ecosystem of microscopic flora and fauna that do more good than harm, so those who wince at the thought of 'creepy crawlies' being fellow travellers should treat them with more respect.

Creepy Crawlies (Mites)

Our most permanent companion, the follicle mite *Demodex folliculorum*, thrives happily in all hairy places including our eyelashes. These fine fellows prevent unwanted particles of skin, bacteria, sebum and other secretions from building up and causing all sorts of problems such as clogged pores. Just think, unless you are devoid of hair, many at this moment are running up and down your eyelashes, keeping them in spick and span condition! A mite is one third of a millimetre long, shaped like a worm so that it can crawl in and out of the narrow cavities between the hair and follicle wall. The male mite is dubiously endowed with a bi-pronged penis on his back and copulates successfully with the female species in our hair follicles! The mind boggles. One or two mites per eyelash is the norm – anything more could lead to a feeling of fullness of the eyelids, itchiness or the sensation of a thriving bordello.

One not too uncommon bed fellow is the scabies mite *Sarcoptes scabiei* which causes scabies. Sufferers itch tremendously and very often the presence of this parasite is wrongly treated with steroids or diagnosed as eczema. The human scabies mite (*Sarcoptes scabiei hominis*) survives only on humans and is just visible to the naked eye. It lives in hairless places where the female forms a burrow in the skin, from whence it can be extricated using a needle. The burrows are visible just beneath the skin, usually at a natural bend or wrinkle. The scabies mite is spread through close contact with an infected person. Some time ago adults were thought to have to perform encounters of the passionate variety to acquire an infestation. However, children can get this by simply sharing beds and bed-clothing. One would know if a scabies mite was in residence because three months after infestation occurred one would be afflicted by day time discomfort and suffer sleepless nights because of itching.

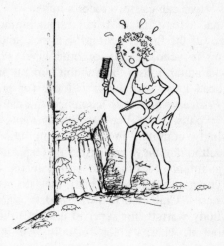

'Don't forget the pan and brush, darling.'

The *Dermatophagoides pteronissinus* dust mite does not take up permanent residence on our bodies but certainly settles comfortably into our beds and other household furnishings. Commonly known as house dust mites, they gobble flakes of dead skin. Although house dust mites are responsible for many allergic responses including asthma, without them the state of the human being does not bear thinking about. Never mind, 'Turn out the lights darling', more a case for, 'Don't forget the pan and brush, darling'. At least the house dust mite is useful, which is more than can be said for bed bugs. Defined as any of several bloodsucking wingless insects of temperate regions that thrive in dirty houses, these 'creepies' suck away at our blood with gusto during nocturnal slumbers. (Personally, we'd recommend sleeping suspended from a chandelier.)

Other mites can migrate from the work place to the body.

People who work with food products can get *Pyemotes ventricosus*, a mite that can cause 'grain itch'; *Tyrophagus casei* mites living on rinds of stored cheese rind cause the 'cheese itch'; and *Glyciphagus domesticus* mites thriving in poor quality sugar can cause 'grocer's itch'.

Add to that a long list of parasites, including ticks and fleas gleaned off the family pet and livestock, and you could be scratching (psychologically or otherwise) well into the night! Lice (singular, louse) that inhabit humans are the body louse, the head louse and the crab louse (or pubic louse). Body lice (*Pediculus humanus humanus*) can cause diseases, particularly typhus. Head lice (*Pediculus humanus capitis*) are surprisingly common in school-going children's hair today, and although they are irritating (especially for the parents or guardians who have to eliminate the critters and their eggs, commonly known as nits), they do not carry any specific diseases. Crab lice (*Pthirus pubis*), like head lice, depend on body warmth for survival and will die within 24 hours without it. These 'crabs' usually live in the pubic region of infected people, and are mainly acquired through sexual contact.

Bacteria

Countless 'good' and 'bad' bacteria (i.e. micro-organisms) live on the dead organic particles of the epidermis and, no matter how much one may try, they can never be eliminated. Even the most hygienic, antiseptic, alcohol treated, scrubbed-four-times-a-day skin will be covered in millions of them. However, take heart – the majority of bacteria living on the skin help to fight invaders and are actually harmless and beneficial. The two main groups of bacteria are the cocci and the diptheroids. Smelly armpits are, incidentally, caused by bacteria decomposing sweat in that region.

Yeast

Yeast is a single celled fungus, which reproduces by budding, i.e. one cell grows out of the parent and breaks free. The most common yeast on the body is of the genus *Pityrosporum*. Living in hair and fatty parts of the skin, such as the scalp and around the nose, is *Pityrosporum ovale*. Another common yeast is *Candida albicans* which can cause the white cobwebby fungus condition known as thrush. This occurs in the bowel and vagina and can occur in the webs of fingers and nails, particularly in people who have constantly wet hands. More recent research has suggested that overgrowth of *Candida albicans* is associated with many health problems including chronic allergy and chronic fatigue (ME – myalgic encephalomyelitis).

Fungi are visiting organisms, which are usually kept at bay by normal skin conditions and human blood, which contains an anti-fungal chemical, as do tears. However, some conditions, such as damp, encourage invasion by dermatophyte fungi. These cause athlete's foot, jockstrap itch and ringworm. Wrong treatment such as antibiotics or fungicides unsuitable for a particular condition can make the situation worse. In addition, the continual use of steroids can lead to an escalation of yeast and fungi populations.

Viruses
These are the smallest live inhabitants of our skin, and are the least studied. Viruses can only reproduce by entering a living cell and 'tricking' it into making more of their own genetic material. One such virus is *Herpes virus hominis*, which causes cold sores, usually in response to low immunity, stress or sunburn. Warts are caused by the *Papova virus*, which stimulates irregular growth of the epidermis. They are benign and if left alone most can disappear within one or two years.

THINGS THAT DAMAGE SKIN
Often we are not aware of the effect of external influences on our health. Unfortunately these influences are everywhere, and, even when we are aware (such as the danger of too much suntanning), our vanity takes over.

Sun

There are many benefits we attribute to the sun: a little exposure makes us feel healthy, helps to stimulate our circulation and activates provitamin D3 in the epidermis, thus enhancing the absorption of calcium. The sun's light and heat rays are essential to life. However, ultra violet rays are disadvantageous as they are the main accelerators of skin ageing. Dermatologists estimate that as much as 80 per cent of the signs of ageing noticeable in our faces are from UV damage, rather than from simply getting older as nature intended. Without sunlight, we might not get our first wrinkles until our sixth or seventh decade. Indeed, skin over the Gluteus Maximus (if you need a clue as to where to find this think upon what you sit – it is not the chair!) is wrinkle free for most of one's life unless one sunbathes nude.

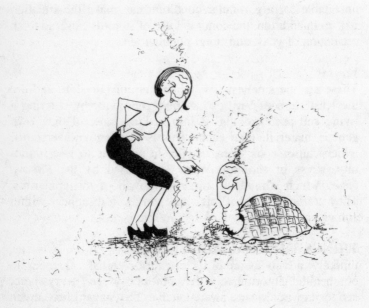

When tortoises begin to give you the wink . . .

Ultra violet rays cause degenerative changes in the deeper layers of our skin, affecting the thickness of our important cushion layer. When the elasticity of this cushion begins to wear, we enter the baggy and drooping era – loose skin under the eyelids (when tortoises begin to give you the wink), to hanging jowls. Hand over the yashmak immediately ... Unfortunately, ultra violet rays are insidious little beggars sneakily breaking down the tissue over many years and suddenly, when it is too late to do anything about it, the collagen and elastin collapses. From this pile of rubble emerges not the dashing phoenix but the skin of an antiquated lizard.

A suntan is simply the body's response to protecting itself. The group of cells in the epidermis of the skin which produce a pigment known as melanin get to work as soon as ultra violet rays start to burn your skin. It may be fashionable to look tanned but if you want to slow down the ageing of your skin either avoid the sun altogether or use a sunblock on the most exposed areas – the face, neck and hands. The first sun care products manufactured provided only UVB filter and did not protect the skin from the photo-ageing capabilities of UVA rays. However, most, if not all, now contain both UVA and UVB filters. Alternatively, try a tinted lotion.

There are three types of UV radiation. UVA, UVB and UVC rays are components, consisting of different wavelengths of sunlight. UVA rays have a longer wavelength and are responsible for only 20-30 per cent of the harmful effects of sun exposure, but penetrate deeper into the epidermis and can cause wrinkling, immunological breakdown and abnormal skin reactions. UVA rays make up about 95 per cent of the total solar UV radiation in summer (depending greatly on climatic and seasonal factors) and cause skin pigment to darken but not become sunburned. UVB rays make up about 5 per cent of the total solar UV radiation around mid-day in summer, and are shorter wavelengths. These rays are mainly responsible for sunburn, which potentially pre-disposes the skin to skin cancer and photo-ageing. UVC rays do not even reach the surface of the Earth because the ozone layer filters them out (despite the 'holes' in it!).

UVB rays are blocked by most window glass and wind-screen glass, but UVA is not, so while you do not get as sunburned behind glass, you still could get long-term damage and skin abnormalities.

An ideal sun care lotion therefore has a balanced UVA/UVB protection and adequate SPF (sun protection factor) which relates to the preparation's UVB screening ability only. (See Sun Care Products, page 61.)

Smoking
There are a great number of oxidative-stress-causing substances with the ability to damage skin, some of which are diesel exhaust particles, nitrogen oxides, ozone, ultra violet rays and cigarette smoke. Despite ultra violet being the most dominant cause of oxidative stress on the human skin, the effect of cigarette smoke is now being looked at as a skin-ageing problem. Cigarette smoke is said to contain two different groups of free radicals, one in the tar substance, the second in the gas. Epidermiological studies have investigated the effect of cigarette smoke on the condition of skin and suggest that smoking is involved in skin disorders and wrinkle formation.

Pollution
Pollution from industrial waste being pumped into the atmosphere is often full of toxic compounds derived from heavy metals. Heavy metals are indeed essential in the body and other life forms for their role in balancing specific chemical processes, but, when excessive amounts of these metals are introduced into the body, disturbing conditions can occur and can lead to disease.

Burns
Any tissue of the body that is damaged by too much heat, radioactivity, electricity or exposure to corrosive chemicals is known as a burn. These can be graded as first, second and third degree burns. A first degree burn involves the surface

epidermis where pain in the affected area can be alleviated by instant flushing with cold water. Sunburn can be a first degree burn. In a second degree burn, blisters form and there is water retention, pain and redness as the whole epidermis and some of the dermis is destroyed. A third degree burn is the most serious, where all skin functions including the nerve endings are lost. Recovery and tissue repair is slow, and when the burn exceeds 70 per cent of the surface area of the body most people die.

Diet and Lifestyle

Both diet and lifestyle contribute to the appearance and state of one's skin. Feeding yourself is not a trivial event as far as your body is concerned, so you should not do so simply out of necessity. Eating correctly – that is, moderate amounts of the right food – can improve health and so improve skin condition too. A balanced diet, correct exercise, plus time for physical and emotional rest, are all essential ingredients for maintaining a healthy body and skin.

Free Radicals

A free radical is a chemical by-product which usually precedes oxygenation, consisting of an atom or a group of atoms containing at least one unpaired electron. Free radicals are oxygen free, unstable and highly reactive. When a free radical takes an electron from one molecule, that molecule becomes unstable and 'borrows' an electron from another molecule, which in turn becomes unstable. Free radicals are believed possibly to contribute to many diseases and disorders. Being highly reactive chemical fragments they can produce irritation to arterial walls and start the arterio-sclerotic process if Vitamin E is missing. They derive from ultraviolet radiation, tobacco smoke, pollution, a thinning ozone layer and poor, high fat diets. Some free radicals also arise naturally in the body. Much of the ageing process is free radical promoted oxidation. Antioxidants, vitamins, minerals and enzymes produced in the body react with these harmful free radicals and normally a healthy body manages to deactivate them (98 – 99 per cent are successfully deactivated). Not all free radicals are unfriendly, for some regulate immune responses and the body's healing mechanisms.

Skin Cancer

Too much sun exposure can result in skin cancer, no matter what the skin pigmentation. A solar keratosis – a pre-cancerous lesion – appears on the skin and looks like a round or irregularly shaped rough scaly surface. There are three most common forms of skin cancer, known as 1) basal cell carcinomas, 2) squamous cell carcinomas and 3) malignant melanomas.

Acne (Acne Vulgaris)

This is a common inflammatory disorder of the sebaceous glands. Acne vulgaris is characterized by the appearance of comedones with papules and pustules. In more severe cases, there are cysts and scars.

3

SKIN CARE PRODUCTS

Skin care products form the largest portion of the cosmetics and toiletries industry, apart from the hair care sector. New technology, new ingredients and the increased use of natural raw materials have led to the development of products that work better and are more aesthetically appealing. The most widely used skin care product is the cream, mainly because its application on the face and body keeps the skin smooth, even disguising a few wrinkles, thereby making a person feel and look good. Humble in its beginnings, it is one of the biggest money-spinners of the cosmetics industry. In that industry, a cream is described as an emulsion. (Not the one you paint the walls with although the concept is the same.) Emulsions are found in various forms, from fluid to very thick, the criterion being decided by the choice of raw materials. An emulsion comprises lipids (the common term for fatty substances), water and an emulsifying agent. An emulsifying factor/agent is incorporated to blend these ingredients together in a stable fashion, the resultant mass being a cream. If an emulsion can be easily poured out of a container it is not referred to as a cream but as a lotion. A sophisticated version of a cream could comprise water, oils, waxes, emulsifiers, preservative, fragrance and colour. Add a 'magic' ingredient or combination of ingredients, package it superbly and look out for the financial deluge.

The majority of cosmetic emulsions are oil and water systems of which there are two important types. The type of emulsion produced depends on the proportions of oil and water used. The oily liquid is known as the oil phase and the water liquid is known as the water or aqueous phase. When the oil phase is dispersed in the aqueous phase the emulsion is referred to as an oil-in-water system and given the symbol o/w. When the water or aqueous phase is dispersed in the oil phase it is referred to as a water-in-oil system and given the symbol w/o. Oil-in-water systems are easily dispersed in water, are readily coloured by water soluble dyes and are less greasy than water-in-oil systems.

Cosmetic scientists have built upon the basic emulsion of a mixture of natural and synthetic waxes and fixed oils (for example, vegetable, animal and mineral oils) to provide different systems for different needs. For example, emulsions are specifically manufactured for: cleansing (including peeling and scrub emulsions), moisturising, night use, day use, for the hands, for the feet, foundation, vanishing and general purpose creams, and skin serums.

There are many substances incorporated into creams and lotions which have excellent humectant (the ability to hold water in a product as well as attract it from the air) properties. One of the oldest reliable humectants is glycerine, which is also used in untangling hair and soothing sore throats. Put some glycerine on a dried up leaf and spread evenly. Wait a few moments and then look at your leaf. It should become smooth. Equal amounts of glycerine and rose water were mixed together to become the first known hand lotion. Other humectants are propylene glycol (used in anti-freeze for cars too!) and sorbitol. When a humectant is part of a moisturising product, it will hold part of the water from the cream for a very long time, while the waxes and oils in the cream will coat the surface of the skin. The combination will make evaporation much more difficult and the skin will benefit by looking and feeling extremely good.

To give the skin the best chance of looking good, three products ought to be used every day. These are, in order of use, **cleansers**, **toners** and **moisturisers**.

CLEANSING PRODUCTS

By cleansing the skin we remove impurities – that is, dirt, a mixture of oil (sebum) and keratinized cells, dust, micro-organisms, make-up and sweat residues, which build up on the skin. The secret is just to take off surface dirt and not the skin's protective layer. Sweating does not clean the skin nor the hair follicle pore through which oil is expelled, although it may clean the openings of the sweat pores. The oil and sweat combine on the skin's surface to form the skin's protective mantle known as the pH balance, which averages at 5.5 – 6.5. (See pH balance, page 27.)

Soap

The oldest and most efficient cleanser is soap and water. However, soap's strong alkalinity can leave the skin feeling very taut and dry and can irritate the eyes or cause rashes depending on its ingredients and the sensitivity of an individual's skin. Soaps described as neutral are in fact generally alkaline, with a pH of about 10 when dissolved in water. Modern soap usually contains a mixture of tallow and nut oil, or fatty acids derived from these substances. Superfatted soaps are those that have unsaponified fat or oil left in the soap, the idea being to leave an oily film on the skin. In liquid soaps, potassium rather than sodium is used. Often synthetic detergents are used, similar to shampoo formulae for liquid soap. Commonly used detergents in these cleansers are sodium laureth sulphate and sodium lauryl sulphate.

Soapless Soap

A silly sounding description – but it is true. Soapwort (*Saponaria officinalis*) is a perennial herb that contains ingredients which lather like a soapy substance but without the drying effect. So, for the soap and water addicts who object to the sting in the face, herein lies the alternative. The only problem is, soapwort can sting the eyes, depending on its concentration level in a product.

Syndet Bar (soap free)

This comprises synthetic detergents and fillers which generally contain no soap at all. Their pH is modified 5.5 to 7.0. The idea behind such products is to formulate a product that would be less irritating to skin. Lanolin and mineral oil may be included in a formula to offer a super-fatted product.

Deodorant Bar

This offers deodorant properties and can include triclosan or triclocarban. The soaps are however, up on the pH scale, reaching 9 to 10, which can cause skin irritation.

Liquid Soaps (detergents)

These products are usually sold in pump dispensers and are designed for hand and face washing. They include detergents such as sodium laureth sulphate, cocamidopropyl betaine and lauramide DEA.

Lipid-free Cleansers

These are products formulated in liquid form to enable cleansing without fats. Their aim is to initiate a lather that can be wiped or rinsed off. Some ingredients may include glycerine, cetyl alcohol, stearyl alcohol and sodium lauryl sulphate.

Foaming Facial Wash

This product is formulated with a small amount of a gentle detergent (mild shampoo type surfactant), plus a good emollient base (skin-softening ingredients), a percentage of humectant and our old friend water. The result is an alternative cleansing medium.

Cleansing Milk (lotion)

This type of product usually has a high water content. As a cleansing medium is designed to remove oil and water-soluble dirt, the formulation need only comprise oils, waxes and water. As a cleanser is applied and quickly removed, it is not necessary for exotic additives to be incorporated. They are added to give marketing appeal. Common ingredients in both creams and lotions include mineral oil, emulsifiers, lanolin, herbal extracts, preservatives, humectants and perfumes. A lotion is a cream (emulsion) with a higher proportion of water.

Cleansing Cream

This was originally known as a cold cream, and was based on one of the oldest known emulsions containing a mixture of natural waxes, such as beeswax, vegetable oils and sodium borate (borax). Cleansing creams are of a thicker consistency than cleansing milk (lotion) as they contain more wax and oil but less water. Some dermatologists say soap and water is just as good as any cleansing cream or lotion, it is cheaper and there is less chance of developing an allergy. However, soap can be more drying and more irritating to the skin. Ingredients are similar to those found in cleansing lotion.

Facial Scrub

This is similar to a cleansing cream but has the addition of a gritty material such as crushed apricot, almond and walnut kernels, which gently abrade the dead top layer of the skin. Other formulations use powdered substances such as corn cob powder while others include polyethylene particles. Some scrubs contain a small amount of detergent while others do not. Care must be taken with scrubs as the scrub material varies in harshness, depending on what type is used, so rather more layers of dead skin may be removed than necessary, resulting in skin sensitivity. Applying facial scrub too often or too vigorously may make the oil glands work overtime and increase the production of oil, the opposite reaction to what was required in the first place, and may also cause epithelial damage.

Exfoliants

These do what the word implies – they exfoliate (flake off) the dead cells of the skin to reveal the underlying fresh layer of skin. Exfoliants are generally formulated to deal with oily skins so are often used by acne sufferers as a replacement for astringents. In fact, exfoliants are, in reality, astringents that have had substances such as witch hazel or salicylic acid added to them to encourage the top layer of skin to flake off. However, such products have been known to contain irritating chemical ingredients.

Eye Make-Up Remover Lotion
This often contains polyglycols (full name is polyethylene glycols) which are helpful in removing oils and waxes used in make-up.

Eye Make-Up Remover Pads
These are pads impregnated with oils, lanolin and, in some instances, a solvent. For hypoallergenic types, pads are soaked in pure mineral oil.

TONING PRODUCTS
A toner (also known as a freshener or astringent – the latter term is often applied to products designed for oily skin) is designed to remove any residue left on the skin after cleansing. This could be make-up, dirt, cream or soap. A good product can help restore the natural acid level of the skin to normal. The differences between toners, fresheners or astringents lies mainly in the percentage of alcohol to water found in any particular product. They all leave the skin with a soothing and cooling sensation and a temporary glowing look.

Toning Lotions
These often contain witch hazel or other astringent products. There may be a high percentage of water to alcohol. Other popular substances are rose water, humectants, herbal extracts, fragrance and preservatives. Non-alcoholic fresheners consist mainly of water with substances such as rose water, sodium borate (borax) and glycerine added.

Tonics (skin fresheners)
These are similar in composition to toning lotion but also contain additives, which suggest healing qualities, such as allantoin, menthol, camphor and azulene. Such additives also give a product a rather delicate pharmaceutical type fragrance and make the skin feel fresh, tight and cool. Tonics are weaker than astringents, containing ingredients such as witch hazel, rose water, orange flower water and many excellent herbal extracts.

Astringents
Astringents contain a high percentage of alcohol. The ingredients used give varying effects such as a tightening sensation of antiperspirant properties and a temporary reduction in pore size. Materials responsible for these effects are organic salts, lower alcohols (no, not the ones from the bottom shelf, simply more gentle versions!), boric acid, alum, menthol and camphor.

MOISTURISING PRODUCTS
A moisturising product should increase the water content of the skin, it should make the skin feel soft and smooth, and it should protect the skin from harmful stimuli. An emollient is any substance or preparation that softens the stratum corneum by increasing its water content, keeping it soft by retarding the loss of its water content. Two mechanisms of emollience present themselves: the prevention of water loss from the skin which allows the build up of water content from within, OR supplementing the skin's water content by attraction of water from the atmosphere by means of a humectant material which serves as a transfer medium. It is the latter action that is popularly described as 'moisturising'. That is why a moisture cream contains a humectant.

Moisturisers come in various forms of textures including milks, lotions, day or night creams and clear gels. Ingredients include mineral oil, water, lanolin, oils of avocado, olive, coconut, safflower, corn and peach kernel, cocoa butter and shea butter, beeswax, sorbitol, polysorbates, Vitamins A, C and E, collagen, elastin, seaweed, preservatives, perfumes, glycerine and petrolatum. Many moisturisers today contain special ingredients known as liposomes, which are apparently able successfully to deliver moisturising ingredients to the epidermis. Other popular substances claimed to improve moisturising efficacy (or to enhance the marketing potential of a product) include ceramides, essential fatty acids, vitamins, collagen, elastin, hyaluronic acid, aloe vera and other botanicals.

Moisturisers should spread easily on the skin and leave it feeling soft, not sticky. How it feels depends on the formulation of the product, i.e. the proportion and quality of the many possible ingredients used. What you choose generally comes down to personal preference, your decision being influenced by the price, packaging, advertising and marketing of any particular product.

Moisturising products generally fall into four main groups, namely body moisturisers, facial moisturisers (that is, day and night preparations), specialised moisturising products and barrier formulae.

Body Moisturisers
Body moisturisers are formulated as lotions, creams, ointments or mousses, although lotions are the most popular preparations. Lotions are generally oil-in-water emulsions with around 75 per cent to 85 per cent water, and are designed to spread more easily than creams or mousse. They may comprise water, mineral oil, stearic acid, petroleum, lanolin and silicone. Richness can be added to a thin emulsion to give a lovely silky feeling by incorporating small amounts of water-soluble gums and some silicones. Humectants such as glycerine and sorbitol, as well as Vitamins A, C and E, and soothing agents such as aloe vera, allantoin or other suitable botanical additives can also be incorporated into moisturisers.

Facial Moisturisers
There are two basic formulae of facial moisturisers and related products: oil-in-water emulsions (which are used in

lighter, day preparations) and water-in-oil emulsions (which are used for the heavier, night preparations). Oil-in-water preparations tend to feel cool and appear non glossy, whereas water-in-oil preparations feel warm and are glossy in appearance. Day moisturising products are usually light in consistency, allowing the product to be easily spread and promoting rapid absorption into the skin. Night moisturisers should be designed to help counter the daily ravages to which the skin is exposed. During sleep, the body does all that it can to restore itself, so a suitable moisturiser that helps to maintain the skin's all important moisture balance is important. *(The ideal time to apply such is perhaps overnight when one could use one of the cheapest and most efficient moisturisers of all – petroleum jelly (petrolatum). Anyone who baulks at your beacon face glistening should be informed you are carrying out a vital (and cheap) exercise in preventing your skin's natural moisture from escaping into the atmosphere. A night cream is much more beneficial when applied a short time before retiring to the arms of Morpheus, otherwise one panders considerably to the vanity of one's pillow. Despite the delights of goodnight kisses from the better half, this unfortunately results in some of the product finding its way onto the skin of the partner. Just let him buy his own!)* The main difference between these moisturising products is simply the additives which can include exotic oils, vitamins, ceramides, fatty acids, collagen, elastin, and herbal extracts.

Facial moisturisers are categorized by skin types. People with oily skins generally choose products that are oil-free or have small quantities of light oil included. Products for normal skins contain moderate amounts of oil and those for dry skin are formulated with even heavier amounts of oil included.

Specialised Moisturising Products

Serums
These are really low viscosity products but with exceptionally high levels of active ingredients such as collagen, elastin,

vitamins and animal complexes. They are used on very dry skin as they can plump it up and give it a radiant appearance.

'Anti-wrinkle' Creams

Any products claiming to contain 'anti-wrinkle' ingredients or referred to as 'youthful skin restorers' or 'wrinkle busters', because countless miracle additives are said to be present, do not cure wrinkles. They do not reverse the ageing process nor do they make wrinkles disappear. In reality such lotions do not penetrate the dermis – very few of the small molecules in a cosmetic product are absorbed into the blood. Officially, manufacturers can only use the term 'anti-ageing' in the title of a product if the text on the label makes it clear that the product can affect only the appearance and 'feel' of the skin. Remember, only collagen injections or cosmetic surgery will get RID of wrinkles. Just to clarify a point here – a hydro-lyzed form of collagen is added to cosmetics as a protein humectant in moisturisers (see **COLLAGEN**, page 116). The injectable collagen comes in a different form, which is suitable for cutaneous and subcutaneous injection.

Eye Creams

Moisturisers manufactured specifically for use around the eyes are known as eye creams, eye balms or anti-wrinkle creams. They are emulsions similar to night creams but contain less oil and are without irritating ingredients such as fragrance materials, which are omitted to prevent eyes stinging. If your face cream causes puffiness under the eyes, a specific eye cream is the answer. A rich emollient applied to the thin absorbent skin of the eyes can increase the fat level in the subcutaneous layer beneath, causing the fat sacs to swell and become puffy. 'Anti-wrinkle eye creams' are simply modified versions of emollient creams and in most instances do not contain a fragrance. Dermatologists gener-ally say eye creams will not prevent wrinkles but may make them less noticeable. Most eye creams contain similar ingredients including beeswax, lanolin, mineral oil, almond and other nut and vegetable oils, cholesterol, lecithin and ascorbyl palmitate. Eye gels often contain soothing extracts, such as cucumber, in a clear gel base.

Vanishing Cream
This is the old name for a moisturising cream.

Foundation Cream
This has many of the same properties as a moisturising cream but is for daytime use so should be non-greasy and matt to enable make-up to be applied on top of it. Much foundation cream also contains emollients, moisturisers and sunscreens. There are also pigmented foundation creams that can contain between 3-25 per cent of pigments, depending on required facial skin shades.

Barrier Preparations
Barrier products are manufactured to protect the hands in much the same way as hand creams. They differ from hand creams by being specially formulated with compounds that prevent certain materials, such as de-fatting solvents, soil, water and dirt, from penetrating the skin. Barrier cream formulae vary depending on their ultimate use. Silicones, petrolatum, zinc oxide, titanium dioxide and beeswax are among common ingredients. Water repellent barrier creams cover the skin with a film that bars water and water soluble agents from entering; oil repellent creams prevent oils from entering the skin.

OTHER HAND PRODUCTS
Hand Moisturisers
These are formulated into lotions or creams. The ingredients used are generally the same as those found in body moisturisers. The hands of the average person take a considerable amount of punishment. If one wants to avoid the gnarled, scaly and inflamed look and opt instead for the 'pale hands I love' scene it is imperative to treat them with respect. Nurture them! Find a product that contains a good emollient and a healing agent such as allantoin, azulene or bisabolol (active

ingredient of chamomile). Petroleum jelly is greasy but an excellent emollient and the addition of silicone derivatives can help the product to be water-resistant. If the hands are in and out of water, then a product with a barrier factor is recommended. Some barrier ingredients are waxes, silicones, petrolatum and mineral oil. Even the idle rich should take note because the many visits to the toilet each day, followed by washing of hands (well, one hopes you do anyway), require emollient recompense. Hand creams can contain emulsifiers, oils, silicone fluid, a humectant such as mannitol, lanolin and water. They should have a pH of between 5 and 8 and should smooth and slide easily into the skin without stickiness, leaving a residual protective film on the skin.

Hand Cleansers
These are alternatives to soap and water. They are manufactured in the form of cream, liquid or gel and contain some of the attributes of a moisturising medium but with a small amount of detergent.

Hand Cleansers (delicate)
For the few people whose hands know little of what is going on in our dirty old world, an emollient milk, cream, lotion or gel should be used. However, a good hand cream is still needed afterwards.

Heavy Duty Hand Cleansers
These are designed for the manual worker whose hands are subjected to well above average grime. For this requirement, there are kerosene-based creams and gels. The kerosene is deodorised and is usually complemented by emollient factors. Some heavy cleansers also contain a detergent ingredient and grit. They are usually recommended in conjunction with a barrier cream.

FOOT PRODUCTS
The poor old feet take our weight all day long and sometimes all night as well. We cover them in cotton, occlusive man-made

fibres and encase them in shoes, boots, Wellingtons, socks and choking tights. We then have the audacity to wonder why we often feel 'foot weary'. Why not give them the pampering they deserve and soak them in a foot-bath for ten to twenty minutes? If boredom sets in, read a recipe book and find out how to make choux pastry! Or watch sport on TV! There are many pleasant ingredients that can be added to a foot-bath. An infusion of fresh herbs like lavender, lime blossom and rosemary added to the water is most reviving. So much so, that domestic animals in the household, as well as the wild fellows (if you have left the window open), may wish to join you.

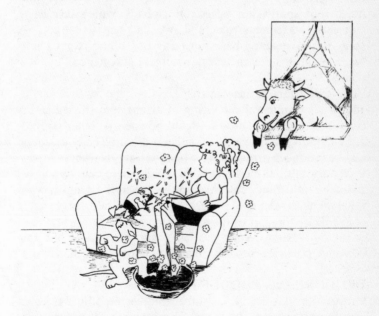

So refreshing it is, that domestic animals in the household, as well as the wild fellows (if you have left the window open), may wish to join you.

Foot Lotions
Lotions specifically formulated for the feet generally contain cooling, soothing anti-inflammatory properties. Ingredients

can include allantoin, azulene, essential oils such as menthol, German and Roman chamomile, sandalwood, peppermint and lavender. Tea tree oil is gaining in popularity due to its anti-bacterial and anti-fungal properties.

Foot Creams
These are suitable for dry skin and should be gently massaged into the dry areas. The ingredients are similar to that of a foot lotion but lie in a richer base (i.e. emulsion) with lower water content.

Foot Sprays
Most foot sprays are based on alcohol, which can carry antiseptic ingredients, essential oils and herbal extracts. A spray is convenient when showering or bathing is not possible. In fact, it is the answer to emergency hygiene.

Foot Talc (talcum powders)
Talc is a soft mineral consisting of magnesium silicate and is used in the manufacture of talcum powder. Another ingredient talcum powder may include is cornflour. Today cosmetic talc has to meet stringent specifications and be asbestos free. If any crystalline silica is present in talc, there may be a small risk of a mild fibrogenic reaction in the user's lungs. Avoid inhalation of talcum powder. Again, foot talc serves as a convenient stop-gap to disguise offensive odours when conventional washing is not available (simply because talc is a convenient carrier of perfume and remains on the skin.)

DEODORISING PRODUCTS
Perspiration (sweat) is the salty fluid secreted by the sweat glands of the skin. Its main function is to regulate body temperature by providing a cooling mechanism through moisture evaporation. Sweat is a mixture of water, amino acids, urea, uric acid, ammonia, lactic acid, glucose, ions and ascorbic acid.

There are two main types of sweat glands: eccrine and apocrine. The eccrine glands are more common than the apocrine glands and are found all over the skin's surface except in the margins of the lips, nail beds of the fingers and toes, pubic areas and eardrums. They empty into an excretory duct that ends as a pore on the surface of the epidermis.

The apocrine glands are found mainly in the armpits, the dark area around the nipples and in the pubic area. Their excretory ducts open into the hair follicles of the skin so they secrete through the same pores as sebum (the human oily substance). Apocrine sweat glands begin to function at puberty and produce a thicker secretion than eccrine glands. They are stimulated under times of emotional stress and sexual excitement. It is believed that human sweat takes on an odour from puberty and it is a possibility that pheromones, the chemical substances secreted by mammals, affect the behaviour of humans too.

Sweat is not offensive when fresh but when it decomposes on the skin's surface it can, to put it mildly, stink. The excreted fatty amino acids start to smell when bacteria act upon it and begin to decompose it. The smell is worsened by the presence of hair that acts as a 'sponge' for the secretions and the consequent attracted bacteria.

The use of antiperspirant and deodorant products has increased greatly in the developed world since the mid-1950s. They are made in the forms of aerosols, roll-ons, sticks, creams, powders and squeeze bottles. The two main active ingredients used in antiperspirants and antiperspirant-deodorants today are aluminium chlorohydrate (ACH) and aluminium zirconium chlorohydrate (AZCH). Although most people believe a deodorant is the same as an anti-perspirant, they do have unique properties. It should be pointed out, however, that while an antiperspirant is also a deodorant, a deodorant is **not** an antiperspirant! This is because aluminium salts contain particular bacteria-halting compounds that control the growth of bacteria. So it's OK for antiperspirant labels to contain the description 'antiperspirant/deodorant' but it is never the other way round.

Deodorants

A deodorant reduces or hides smell from the axillary regions by using a perfume or an anti-microbial agent, which helps to neutralise the unpleasant odour of decomposing bacteria by inhibiting the growth of such microorganisms.

Lichen (such as alpine lichen, which is found suspended from tree branches in the Alps) can be used in deodorants but is a skin sensitizer. The active ingredient of alpine lichen and related species is usnic acid.

Antiperspirants

An antiperspirant works by limiting the secretion of sweat in the armpits by helping to block the little pores where the sweat comes out. Compounds used in antiperspirants are aluminium salts or zirconium salts, a bactericide and a fragrance. Remember, deodorants and antiperspirants are complementary to good hygiene and should not be used instead of a really good bath or shower.

Vaginal Deodorants

Some women who have used these products (usually in the form of powders and aerosols) designed to prevent 'feminine odour' have suffered bladder infection and irritation, swelling, boils, itching and rashes after application. Doctors generally recommend simple soap and water to do the job more safely and efficiently. Ingredients in vaginal deodorants include perfume, glycerides, propellants, antibacterials, myristate and polyoxyethylene derivatives among others.

SHAVING PRODUCTS

Alexander the Great made shaving fashionable among the Greeks around the fourth century BC. By shaving, there was no longer any possibility of the beard being used as a convenient tool for someone to grip firmly onto while slitting the bearded one's throat or as a help in total decapitation. (He actually ordered his soldiers to shave as a precaution against this very action.) Shaving products, men's fragrances and hair preparations specifically designed for men are the most popularly purchased of all the toiletries made for men. Shaving products have been around in various forms for many years and are used as part of a daily routine (or chore). Indeed, if one did not shave from the onset of puberty until middle age (55 years) one would have a beard of around 27.5 feet (8 metres)! The rate of hair growth of the beard is similar to that of the eyebrows and body hairs (not including pubic and armpit regions), a rate of about 0.3-0.4 millimetres per day.

Use of the correct shaving products and the correct methods (that is, not doing it while driving to work) determines a good or bad shave. Preparing the face by wetting with warm water allows the hairs to soften. The angle, sharpness and pressure of a blade are all important, as is the application of a cream or foam to help the blade glide. Today's electric razors, however, cut out the need for much of the above.

Of course, nowadays women shave too and use shaving creams and gels.

Shaving Creams (lather)
Shaving creams that lather are designed to reduce razor burn. They are predominantly made up of sodium and potassium soaps. The latter generate lather bubbles better than sodium based soaps. Lather keeps the facial hair moist and lubricated during shaving. Shaving creams contain ingredients including coconut oil, diethanolamide, dispersants, fatty acids, water, perfume, menthol, camphor, isopropyl myristate and alcohol.

Aerosol Shaving Foams
These generally consist of water, lauryl alcohol, stearic acid, coconut fatty acids, triethanolamine, perfume and preservatives, plus a butane propellant. These are easy to use, producing an instant lather. Aerosol shaving foam is similar but not quite the same as a mousse.

Shaving Gel

This product is similar to shaving foam but is separated from the butant propellant by a piston to produce a clear gel. Gels are thought to produce a better shave because of their surfactant (wetting agent) content. These agents penetrate hair, making it swell with moisture and so uncurl and straighten. This makes the hair easier to cut and also helps prevent infection from ingrown hairs and razor bumps.

Shaving Oils

These products are effective as they drastically reduce the glide of the razor blade as it passes over the skin. They usually contain silicone oils with low coefficients of friction.

Shaving Creams (brushless)

These are similar to cold creams but have added lubricants and contain water, stearic acid, mineral oil, lanolin, preservatives and thickeners.

Pre-electric Shaving Lotions

These products are designed for dry shaving to remove a film of moisture from the face and beard, depositing a film of emollient to improve razor cutting. For successful shaving with an electric razor it is better for the facial hair to be stiff and dry. The lotion generally contains alcohol, which is antiseptic and gives a slightly astringent feel.

Aftershave Lotions

These alcohol- or ethanol-based lotions are made to relieve some of the discomfort of shaving and generally consist of ingredients that cool and refresh the skin and close pores, so protecting it from bacterial invasion. Ingredients include glycerine, water, a humectant, emollient, menthol (for its cooling effect), colour and perfume. Alum or witch hazel may be added for their astringent-styptic (i.e. contracting the blood vessels and tissues) effect, as too might allantoin help heal razor cuts quickly. An anti-bacterial ingredient may also be used to prevent infection. Non-alcoholic aftershave lotion is similar in make up to that of hand lotion, which can in fact be used instead.

Aftershave Creams (balm)
These are designed to relieve the discomfort of shaving by soothing and cooling the skin, and contain only a low level of alcohol (or none at all) as it can irritate sensitive skins. They are emulsions with emollients, a humectant, plant extracts, fragrance and essential oil constituents such as menthol or azulene.

BABY PRODUCTS
Lotions
In our continuing search for skin as smooth as a baby's bottom it is easy to forget that after infancy, through puberty to the final decrepit stage, 'baby products' are incapable of producing baby-type skin on anyone except babies. Baby lotions based on a high water content make excellent cleansing lotions because they are light in texture and soothing. They generally contain humectants, mineral oils, anti-microbials, lanolin, emulsifiers, preservatives, antioxidants, cetyl alcohol, thickeners, and much use is made of the sorbitan ester types of ingredients.

Protective Creams
Protective creams do as the word suggests – they create a barrier on the baby's skin to prevent chapping and allow healing as they contain useful ingredients such as zinc oxide, petroleum jelly, silicones and lanolin.

Baby Oil
This is used to stop the baby squeaking! Actually, it is a cleansing and protecting medium for babies. Baby oils can contain mineral and vegetable oils, lanolin derivatives, isopropyl palmitate, polyethylene dilaurate and perfume.

BATH PRODUCTS
Bath products are used not only to clean the body; many are designed to impart a pleasant aroma and soft feel to the skin.

Bath products also soften the water and so prevent a hard-water scum from forming around the bath at water level.

Floating Bath Oils

Due to their chemical composition, oils float on top of water. Consider an oil slick! If the product does not contain a detergent factor, the floating oil will not move smoothly across the water but can produce large globules which then adhere to the bather's skin, making it feel uncomfortably greasy. There will also be the drawback of an oily rim around the bath, and, should the bather decide to stand in the bath while towelling dry as the water drains away, the risk of sliding on the bath's oily residue is rather obvious. The practice of adding a few drops of an essential oil to a vegetable or mineral oil (correct description being a fixed oil) is foolhardy to say the least. Water and oil by their natures DO NOT MIX: oil will float on the water's surface. A pleasant product would include an oil soluble surfactant to enable the oil to form a continuous film over the water. Ingredients found in this type of product are mineral oil, isopropyl myristate, emollients, fatty acid esters, castor oil, vegetable oil and fragrance (as much as 10 per cent, so beware, perfume sensitive people).

Soluble Bath Oils

These are also described as emulsifying bath oils and are designed to disperse into the bath water. They are transparent emulsions and are available as concentrates, comprising fragrance, surfactant, water and sometimes alcohol.

Blooming Bath Oils

We are not being rude. Blooming bath oils, also described as dispersing bath oils, comprise oil, an emollient ingredient, a surfactant and fragrance. When added to the bath water they disperse with a milky effect. The performance of a soluble bath oil and a dispersing type is to deposit oil on the skin. However, when 'dispersed', less oil adheres to the skin.

'Eye-catching' Bath Oils

These bath oils are not formulated for extra benefit to the skin but are designed for consumer appeal. They comprise two to three layers which disperse and foam in the bath water. The layers are of different colours which, on dispersion, produce an eye-catching change in colour. A two-layer product could contain, for example, ingredients such as sodium laureth sulphate, mineral oil, hexylene glycol, propylene glycol, dicaprylate dicaprate, perfume, preservatives and colours.

Bath Essences

Bath essences are formulated to convey fragrance to the bath water. This provides an excellent opportunity to spend quality time soaking in an aromatic bath. Ingredients used are similar to those used in soluble and blooming bath products, although alcohol is often employed to give the perfume a stronger aroma.

Silicone-based Bath Oils

These are for people who dislike the oily film of bath oils. The glycolcopolymers employed in these products leave the skin feeling velvety soft without the tackiness associated with fixed oils.

Bath Salts

Bath salts soften the bath water. The most popular ingredient is sodium sesquicarbonate. Other ingredients are borax and trisodium phosphate. To make the product more effervescent, ingredients such as citric acid and sodium bicarbonate are incorporated. The addition of fragrance and colour make an attractive product.

Bath Cubes

The same ingredients as bath salts are utilised in bath cubes but the salts are ground down to a powder and combined with starch and a binding agent. Often a detergent factor is included, such as sodium lauryl sulphate. Other ingredients include fragrance, preservative and colour.

Effervescent Bath Tablets and Balls

These tablets rapidly disintegrate in the bath water. The favourite ingredients for such products are sodium bicarbonate plus citric or tartaric acids, sodium sesquicarbonate, perfume, preservative and colour.

Foaming Bath Products (i.e. bubble baths)

Foaming bath gels, foam baths, crème baths, herbal baths and shower gels are formulated from similar ingredients. The products are designed to cleanse, leaving a pleasant fresh after feel and soft velvety skin. Adults and children enjoy using these products for the fun of creating copious quantities of foam and generally for making bathing a special event of the day. Foam should occur in any temperature and in both hard and soft water, should not collapse the moment soap is added to the water yet should not be too stable as to make it hard to get rid of down the plug-hole. Their only use is as a fun product, although they do prevent a scum ring from forming around the bath. Ingredients include a primary detergent, a secondary detergent with milder properties, good foaming and foam stabilising ability. The milder secondary detergent can help mitigate any irritating effect of the primary detergent. Added to these ingredients are a viscosity regulator, pH adjusting ingredient, preservative, colour and fragrance. Herbal, fruit and seaweed extracts and essential oils are popular additives. A label could read: sodium laureth sulphate, cocamidopropyl betaine, cocoglucoside, hydrogenated castor oil, distearate sodium, parfum, citric acid. Additives such as marigold, chamomile, horse chestnut extracts, grapefruit, fruit extracts, vitamin E, essential oils and colour are commonly used.

Shower Gels

Easier to use than soap, shower gels are highly viscous liquids and extremely popular. As they are used all over the body the ingredients have to be chosen carefully for mildness because of possible contact with vulnerable areas such as the eyes. A popular primary detergent is sodium laureth sulphate, a secondary one being sodium laureth sarcosinate (it is milder). Foaming and stabilising ingredients may be provided by the betaines (types of surfactants) and beneficial conditioning properties provided by a quaternary ammonium compound (this is a cationic surfactant – these are good conditioners and have a bactericidal action). Additives may include proteins, vitamins, seaweeds, fixed oils such as vitamin E oil, apricot kernel, herbal extracts, fruit extracts or essential oils, each additive with its own USP (unique selling point).

Foaming Bath Oils
These products are extremely difficult to formulate as the addition of a reasonable amount of an oily emollient has the capacity to depress the foaming effect. A foaming bath oil is really a compromise of a foam bath and a bath oil.

OTHER PRODUCTS
Sun Care Products
A moderate amount of exposure to the sun makes us feel healthy and happy; deprivation of it can lead to a type of winter depression known as Seasonal Affective Disorder (SAD). Too much can lead to premature ageing and skin cancer. A balanced exposure to sunlight is therefore essential to good health. To allow us some time in the sun, yet to prevent the damage from ultra violet (UV) rays, specific sunscreen products have been formulated. The UVA and UVB rays which can damage our skin are discussed in detail on page 35. Sunscreens are divided into two types: chemical sunblocks and physical sunblocks. Chemical sunblocks, such as PABA (para amino benzoic acid) esters and isopropylbenzyl salicylate contain molecules that absorb the radiant light energy, while physical sunblocks (such as titanium dioxide, zinc oxide, magnesium silicate and kaolin) place a coating on the skin that reflects sunlight.

An ideal sunscreen lotion should contain a balanced UVA/UVB protection factor and adequate SPF (sun protection

factor which relates to the preparation's UVB screening
ability only). A product labelled SPF20, for example, means
that the sun protection factor enables a person to stay in the
sun without getting burnt 20 times longer than if the skin was
unprotected. However, the person could still get heatstroke. A
good combination of ingredients in a sun care product could
also include the non-toxic and non-irritating substances
ultrafine titanium dioxide and ultrafine zinc oxide, which
have become widely accepted for UV screening among
cosmetic and toiletry manufacturers.

Research into new ingredients continues rapidly, and
formulae are changing alongside new discoveries. Studies
have even revealed that pansy extract and green coffee
extract may be good news as they can complement synthetic versions with their ability to absorb ultra violet
signals.

Even if you use a sun protection cream regularly it is
still not good for your health to lie in the sun. While the
use of sunscreens with a high protection factor (SPF15-50)
can extend our solar exposure by many hours, even to all
day exposure, the long term biological consequences are
undetermined. Opinions vary, but it will only be when
the teenagers of today are in their forties, fifties or
sixties that the real benefit of high SPF sunscreens will be
realised.

Sunscreen products are available on the market in the form
of gels, ointments, emulsions, sticks, mousses and aerosols.

After-sun Products
For those of you who still manage to get sunburnt, soothing,
cooling lotions containing ingredients such as bisabolol,
essential oil of lavender, lanolin, menthol (cooling), a
humectant and herbal extracts are formulated to return fats
and moisture to the skin. Allantoin, aloe vera, Vitamin A and
calamine, with their soothing and healing properties, could
also be incorporated. After-sun products can be used even if
you do not get burnt – they soothe, moisturise and maintain
the skin's condition.

Tinted Lotions
Be assured that using a tinted lotion or cream is absolutely
fool-proof if you want the tanned look. But make sure you
choose a product that suits your skin, along with a tan
colour which blends in and does not go on like a heavy
foundation cream. Remember that a fake tan simply stains
the skin and does not protect it against UVA or UVB rays,
although there has been a suggestion by researchers that the
staining ingredient known as DHA (dihydroxyacetone) may
possibly give UVA protection. However, as this has not yet
been clinically proven, stay in the shade or use an additional
sunscreen. Within a few hours of applying an artificial
tanning lotion containing DHA, the skin will darken and the
tan will last for the life of the epidermis.

*Maurene writes: Since understanding the effect of ultra
violet rays I have used an artificial tan lotion and I am often
asked: 'Have you been on holiday? You look so tanned!' Well
the last word is yours but have a good peek at the skins of
outdoor workers and if you want to look gnarled and brown
then just get under that star!*

*During my career as an airhostess I managed to catch a bit
more sun than advisable during a stopover in Karachi. Being
an ardent curry fiend and an incessant chatterer on the
subject I was invited to the hotel's kitchin to meet the chef. He
was extremely affable and more than pleased to know I was
doing justice to his curries at breakfast, luncheon and dinner.
He showed me many spices and gave tips on blends and
procedures. A few nights later, no doubt due to the lack of
noise, the head waiter asked where I was, and one of the crew
explained my sunburn predicament. As we were about to
leave the hotel the next day, the chef appeared to bid farewell
and gave me a little bottle containing some perfumed liquid to
apply to my burning parts. I applied some to my face and
neck which were indeed scarlet, and worked during the trip in
the galley in case the passengers thought I was totally
dedicated to alcohol both on and off duty! I have never found
out what that soothing lotion was, the only side effect being
that it made my skin a very bright yellow which lasted two*

*days and earned me the nickname of 'haldi (turmeric) chops'
for ages afterwards. (Turmeric is used by people in India for
healing purposes – indeed, the poor person's answer to
antibiotics.)*

Masques

Masques are formulated to remove dead cells, to clean,
soothe, soften, nourish, tighten and brighten the face. Dermatologists say there is no evidence to suggest that any
cosmetics can shrink pores, while wrinkles can really only
be removed by surgery or diminished by injections of
collagen. Masques do, however, relax a person and induce a
light, fresh feeling afterwards. Clay face masques generally
contain glycerine, water, siliceous earth, kaolin, acacia,
waxes, certain oils, titanium oxide and other ingredients.
Papaya (which is, incidentally, used as a tenderiser on steak)
is an excellent natural ingredient as it eats protein, i.e. it
devours dead skin cells. Bentonite, a white clay, is commonly found in masques to thicken and soak up sebum on
the face to stop it from shining.

Hydrocolloid Masques

These are formulated from gums and humectants. They have
tremendous consumer appeal due to added ingredients such as
avocado and almond oil, zinc oxide, honey and oatmeal.
Again, they leave a pleasant after feel of slightly tightened
and smooth skin.

Wax Masques

Wax masques comprise paraffin wax, into which petroleum
jelly and/or beeswax is dissolved. Applied warm to the skin,
they have an occlusive action preventing transepidermal
water loss. On removal, a rich moisturising medium is
applied and the skin can feel smooth with an excellent
emollient effect.

*Maurene writes: A company I worked for when I first
came into the cosmetics industry required, for a skin care
range, a masque suitable for mature skin. As I have had*

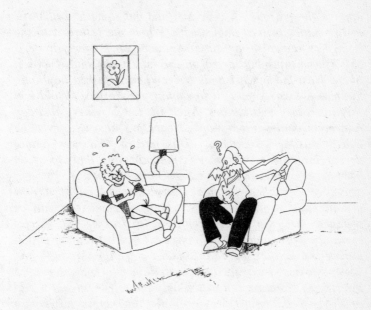

The masque had dried on the moustache and it looked like a frost-laden Christmas tree.

mature skin for longer than I care to remember I had immense fun trying out different types. The best was a delightful blend of natural materials that made the skin extremely soft but, while on the face, turned a silvery white. One Sunday I had a complete pamper – I ran a bath to which I added some fragrant herbs, applied the masque to my face and, to complete my paradise, went to extract a glass of wine from the sitting room where my beloved sat, by now agape, wondering what I had on my face. Fascinated with my explanation about how it cleansed and softened my skin, he asked if there was any more so that he too could apply it. I gave him the remainder and went to wallow in the tub. A little later my daughter Andrea burst into the bathroom saying she couldn't sit in the lounge any longer without exploding with mirth as not only had my beloved applied the masque all over his face but some had adhered to his rather profuse moustache. When she returned to the lounge to replenish my glass she came back nearly hysterical. The masque had dried on the moustache and it looked like a frost-laden Christmas tree. When he asked how long the masque was supposed to remain on the face, I told him fifty instead of ten minutes. After all, fun is fun. To this day Andrea crumples into a helpless cackling mass whenever the word 'masque' is uttered. (This masque did not contain drying ingredients therefore lengthening the time spent on his face did no harm. It did them both good too.)

Before I studied cosmetic chemistry, I bought a new product that professed to tighten and smooth the skin. It sounded like a Cinderella treatment for making that special evening a spectacularly self confident one. I tried the potion during the daytime and it did indeed make the skin tight and young-looking. I was invited out to dinner by a gentleman to the type of restaurant of which only the self-indulgent would approve. I thought I would apply the magic elixir that evening and so impress him with my youthful looks. All went well until the middle of the main course when I noticed my friend's surreptitious glances towards me. These rapidly changed to stares of disbelief and then to wide-eyed horror. Finally he leant forward and in a startled voice said: 'What the blazes is happening to your face?' I was mortified. Before I could gather my wits he croaked: 'Your face is breaking up.' I bolted into the ladies and in the mirror there reflected something which could have won an Oscar in a horror film. The magic elixir had dried out completely and was peeling off in huge cobwebby layers. Bits hung off my nose, my cheeks and forehead. I hadn't felt anything, possibly because I had previously applied a thin layer of moisturising cream. As I finished washing it off, I envisaged my escort's face and fell over the sink, screaming with laughter, much to the alarm of a dear old lady who had come in to use the facilities in the way they were intended. My visibly shaken friend eventually saw the funny side, albeit after five brandies.

Massage Cream

A massage cream requires good skin slip, which means the ability to withstand being rubbed on the skin, yet not being absorbed, otherwise the skin can be slightly irritated. A good massage cream comprises certain occlusive ingredients, such as petrolatum, mineral wax and mineral oil. It may also contain emollient ingredients such as cocoa butter, vegetable oils and silicones. If the product used is based on totally occlusive ingredients, it is a good idea to bath or shower after the massage. The reason for this is that occluding the skin for some time can have an adverse effect on its ability to eliminate waste products.

4

LEGISLATION REGARDING COSMETIC PRODUCTS

Cosmetic product safety legislation is complex but highly necessary to safeguard public health and to help manufacturers stay on the right track. In 1976 an EEC Council Directive was introduced, harmonising cosmetic safety legislation among the European Economic Community. Many amendments including the requirement for full ingredient listing on products have subsequently occurred, and consolidating all previous directives are the latest UK regulations known as The Cosmetic Products (Safety) Regulations 1996. (Note: This is the Criminal Law. The Consumer Protection Act and other laws provide for remedies in civil actions.) Basically these regulations limit the nature and strength of many ingredients used, and each new product destined to be launched upon the public has to be formally certified by a recognised safety assessor.

Cosmetics are not supposed to be marketed to resemble medicines, but 'borderline' products between medicines and cosmetics do appear. Officially, medicines alter the function of the skin or treat a medical condition whereas cosmetics temporarily affect only how it looks or feels. Should there be any doubt as to a product's status the Medicines Control Agency, which regulates medicinal products for human use in the UK, will be able to advise. Consumers confused by marketing jargon could consult a dermatologist before purchasing a £300 pot of face cream, or dig into the laws on advertising – the realm of the Advertising Standards Authority.

Aromatherapy products come under different regulations (i.e. General Product Safety Regulations 1994) so are only described as cosmetic products if they are intended to be placed in contact with the external body surfaces as previously mentioned, and are intended to clean, perfume, change the appearance of, protect, keep in good condition or to correct body odours. The Aromatherapy Trades Council can provide valuable advice. Again, this is only regarding Criminal Law; the Consumer Protection Act and others provide for remedies in civil action where harm is claimed.

A cosmetic ingredient is any synthetic or natural substance used in manufacturing a cosmetic product. An international system has been developed for the labelling of ingredients used in cosmetic products. This system is basically an inventory of cosmetic ingredients and is known as the INCI (International Nomenclature of Cosmetic Ingredients) system, which was produced by a European trade group working closely with an equivalent organisation from the United States. The aim was to establish an international system so that consumers from any EU country or the USA would be able to recognise instantly any ingredient that may be listed on a product manufactured in a different member country. For example, instead of using 'water' or its equivalent in many different languages, a standardised 'aqua' (INCI name) is used instead. 'Beeswax' is known as 'cera alba' (INCI name) throughout Europe and the USA. In the absence of any INCI name, a chemical name, European Pharmacopoeia name or other recognised identifying name can be used.

The INCI names for cosmetic ingredients are mandatory and are the only names that can be used in the EU and USA (and some other countries) for labelling. There are many technical names for any substance, which explain its chemical structure, but these are often too long to put on a cosmetic product. There are also trade names that may appear on some labels.

Cosmetic manufacturers in New Zealand, Australia and South Africa follow the INCI naming system for ease of clarity and acceptability in Europe or the USA, but it is not compulsory for them to do so. There is a general worldwide acceptance of this INCI labelling system.

Animals and Cosmetic Testing

Skin care products can make our lives much more enjoyable by making us look and feel good. However, it would be unwise to buy any product, be it for eating, drinking, gardening, washing up or applying to the skin, without feeling reasonably sure that one was not going to suffer nasty effects that could range from mild irritation to a serious skin disease. To ensure this, companies manufacturing cosmetics are required by law to establish potential hazards to consumer health as well as to protect the workers involved in their production. This means that many of the ingredients in personal care products such as skin creams, soaps, deodorants, shampoos and toothpastes, as well as perfumes and colour products (e.g. lipstick and eyeshadow), must be tested. In earlier years this typically involved some testing on animals. The latest EU regulations say that no one may supply to consumers a cosmetic product or any cosmetic ingredient that has been tested on animals after 1st January 1998. A report by the European Commission in 1997 recognised that work still needed to be done on alternatives, so the ban was deferred to 30th June 2000.

Any cosmetic companies that claim their products have not been tested on animals (e.g. where 'cruelty free' or 'not tested on laboratory animals' is found on the label) may be misleading buyers into believing that these products have no connection at all with the use of animals. This is often not the case, because many frequently used ingredients have already been individually tested on animals, possibly because they have additional uses of an entirely different kind. You may find that manufacturers also say that, although a material they are using for cosmetic purposes has not been tested for cosmetic purposes by themselves, it may well have been tested in other industries such as the food or pharmaceutical industries. There is therefore a regulation which stipulates that any reference to testing on animals in the labelling or advertising of a cosmetic product must state clearly whether the tests carried out involved the cosmetic product itself or its ingredients or both. Any 'reference' includes any emblem, trademark, picture signs and so on that refer to animal testing.

FRAME (the Fund for the Replacement of Animals in Medical Experiments, located in Nottingham) cautions against relying on the use of labelling on the basis of products containing only new mixtures of old and tested ingredients, and recommends that 'the sensible way forward is to develop and validate reliable alternative methods for regulatory acceptance'.

One example of an ingredient test performed on an animal is the Draize eye test, when the chemical under test is put into a rabbit's forced-open eye. Another test for discovering the comedo-producing potential of ingredients used in the formulation of skin care products uses the external ear canal of a rabbit. The substance being tested is applied once daily, and after the fourteenth application the animals are killed and cross sections of the canal evaluated. Another test is the Draize skin test where the ingredient is applied to rabbit skin. Even when it is simply a sample of blood being taken, all animals used in tests have to be killed at the end of the tests. However, several alternatives to this particular test have been developed but none is considered suitable as a complete replacement to the Draize eye test, and other methods are still being sought.

History of Alternatives: the Three Rs
In 1959, two English researchers, Lillian Russell and Rex Burch, proposed the concept of replacement, reduction and refinement (now known as the Three Rs) as a way to make bio-medical research more humane. They suggested that

scientists in their experiments should always try to:

1. **Replace** the use of higher animals (e.g. mammals) with
    lower organisms (e.g. bacteria) or non-animal methods
    (e.g. tissue culture).
2. **Reduce** the numbers of animals required to an unavoid-
    able minimum; and
3. **Refine** the experiments to minimise the pain or distress
    experienced by any animals which have to be used.

The Three Rs now form the basis of laws such as the Animals
(Scientific Procedures) Act 1986 in the UK and the European
Directive 86/609/EEC, which control the use of animals in
laboratory experiments. Points of interest are:

1. The EC Cosmetic Directive 76/768 EEC 1993 sought to
    ban the use of animals in cosmetics testing from 1998,
    but ONLY for those tests where alternative methods
    have been scientifically validated. It is now UK law that
    no cosmetic products or ingredients can be tested on
    animals in the UK. However, this ban applies only to
    testing carried out in the UK. If a cosmetic manufactur-
    ing company wants to use a particular new ingredient, in
    order to satisfy UK law it will still need to conduct tests
    on animals, but the testing will be done in another
    country! The European Commission hopes eventually to
    ban testing of finished cosmetics in all its EU member
    states.

2. The Seventh Amendment to the 1976 EC Cosmetic
    Directive is a very complex issue, but basically it
    proposes that there be a marketing ban for cosmetics
    containing ingredients, or combinations of ingredients,
    tested on animals only when there are alternative
    forms of testing available. It proposes that when
    manufacturers label products 'not tested on animals' it
    will be acceptable only if the manufacturer and its
    suppliers have not carried out (or got anyone else to

do so) any animal testing on products or ingredients.

3. In all cases, the United Nations Regulations and the general European Union regulations on chemicals take precedence over the cosmetic regulations.

4. It is illegal to manufacture or import into Europe any chemical that does not have an EINECS or ELINCS number. The only way to obtain this registration is to prove the safety of that raw material and the only accepted way is by animal testing. Therefore, new raw materials are not usually tested specifically for cosmetic purposes unless that is the only area in which they are going to be used.

5. Some alternative tests (three in all) have been accepted in the US for testing the corrosiveness of chemicals, and two of these, as well as a test for phototoxicity, have been accepted by the EU.

FRAME and other anti animal testing organisations are working in conjunction with some of the larger pharmaceutical companies constantly searching for new alternatives to animal testing. The Dr Hadwen Trust is a medical charity, which, it says, benefits people as well as animals as its scientists develop and apply non-animal techniques in a wide range of medical fields. Some companies say they use only ingredients accepted as suitable before 27th September 1976 when the Cosmetic Directive of the European Union came into force. Their advertising literature says they do not use new ingredients because they feel these are most often tested on animals, and there are enough usable 'traditional' ingredients around already. However, they would consider using new ingredients when acceptable alternatives to animal testing are verified and made available.

The Humane Research Trust promotes alternatives to animals in medical research generally, and they have been involved in finding alternatives to the Draize eye test. They are also seeking to establish better non-animal testing procedures for detergents.

The safety testing of new cosmetics is one of the areas most readily open to using non-animal methods. Tests, which will hopefully replace the use of living animals for detecting potential eye and skin irritants, are at an advanced stage of development. Some companies already use *in vitro* methods (e.g. cell cultures, bacteria and hen's eggs) as pre-screens before carrying out any animal experiments.

Non-animal alternatives which have been approved by authorities such as the World Health Organisation include physico-chemical methods, for example, high performance liquid chromatography (HPLC), a method which can be used for separating the individual chemicals present in mixtures, which is now used to analyse insulin for impurities. Previously, the purity of each new batch of insulin produced had to be tested on mice.

Mathematical and computer modelling techniques are used to help predict the possible biological effects of chemicals, and computer assisted drug design can help in designing new medicines and other products. Lower organisms such as fungi, bacteria, algae and plants are being used as they have less well-developed nervous systems than vertebrates and are less likely to suffer pain. For example, yeast is being used in tests to detect substances that might cause skin damage in the presence of light (phototoxins). Vertebrates, too, in their early stages of development, can be used – they do not then have a sufficiently developed nervous system that allows pain. Chicken embryos, tadpoles and rat foetuses are being used in tests being developed for identifying chemicals that damage the developing foetus.

Tissues, cells and whole organs can now be kept alive for more than 24 hours in the laboratory in a solution of special nutrients. Cells from organs such as the liver and kidney can be grown in culture, and the effects of chemicals upon them can be investigated. Cell cultures are widely used in developing and screening new medicines and vaccines, and for testing products – including cosmetics – for toxicity.

Human volunteers are used to confirm the safety and efficacy of new cosmetic products, for example in skin patch testing. Where there is already sufficient evidence that a product is not harmful, the skin of human volunteers rather than animals is used to test for possible irritancy of cosmetics. The material under test is incorporated in a large sticking plaster that is applied to the skin.

A potentially very useful alternative method involves a laboratory-grown three-dimensional human skin equivalent tissue composed entirely of metabolically and mitotically active dermal and epidermal cell layers. It is used to assess reactions from a variety of environmental conditions, UV light, cosmetics, drugs and micro-organisms, leading to a wide range of symptoms and diseases from irritation or allergic responses to virulent forms of skin cancer. Human skin cells from various patients are seeded onto a nylon mesh, the co-culture consisting of cells of neonatal foreskin fibroblasts. After four weeks, the epidermal keratinocytes are seeded onto the three dimensional dermis. The dermis is made using dermal fibroblasts mixed with nutrients, vitamins and strands of collagen protein. After 30 days of being stimulated by nutrients including glucose and growth hormones, the new skin has become a replica of human skin. This method has been accepted by the US and Canadian Department of Transportation for clarifying corrosive chemicals.

FRAME has also developed a multi-layer model of the epidermis of human skin in its laboratory at the University of Nottingham, with which it has a close association. The model is principally used to evaluate chemicals that cause skin irritation.

A number of cosmetic companies use specialised products that come in kit form, and contain disks of skin tissue, which are then used for a variety of tests without harm to an animal.

It seems unlikely though, that there will ever be a total end to testing cosmetic ingredients on animals, because many of the ingredients used in cosmetics such as ultra violet filters and preservatives are also used in medicines. Animals still have a vital role to play in finding cures for human diseases.

5

NATURAL COSMETICS

An astounding sum is invested in the marketing of natural skin care products, and the impact on the consumer is unbelievable. There is continual pressure from television commercials, health shop literature, in-store promotions, leaflets, glossy magazines, sharp-shooting sales people, glamorous therapists and more, to buy, buy, buy and 'go for natural'. Among the countless adjectives they use to drive the message home you'll find *gentle*, *natural*, *tranquil*, *organic*, *traditional* – all intended to woo the customer with the rewards of nature's delightful goodies. The aromas alone can conjure up visions of forests and green meadows brimming with health-giving herbs, sweet scented blossoms and intoxicating floral delights. In fact it's clever 'green' marketing, playing on our own urge to reduce the daily stresses, that impels us to break our necks in pursuit of Mother Nature – a treacherous old bat at times, make no mistake! (Ever smelled the natural odour of a skunk or burnt animal after a natural thunderstorm?)

In the cosmetics world, 'natural' is a grey area because even ingredients from a natural source have to be processed in some way before reaching the customer. What needs to be defined is the degree of permissible processing, and as yet there is no legislation or regulatory guideline controlling the use of the word 'natural' in cosmetic products, apart from the general laws laid down by the Advertising Standards Authority. That's why, today, product ingredients fall loosely into four main areas: natural ingredients, synthetic ingredients,

nature identical ingredients and ingredients obtained from
animals. Generally speaking, **natural ingredients** are those
which have been extracted from natural sources. **Synthetic
ingredients** are chemically synthesized substances that are
generally not known to occur in nature. **Nature identical
ingredients** are the same as those that come from parts of
living plants but which have been produced by chemical
reaction rather than actual extraction. **Animal ingredients**
may be procured by killing the animals, or from waste
products of carcasses slaughtered for the meat, or from
by-products such as lanolin. The strong animal odours of
musk (from the musk deer), ambergris (from the sperm
whale) and civet (from glands of the civet cat) were used
much by men in the sixteenth century.

In this war of words between natural and synthetic, the
governing factor is the cost to the consumer. It *is* possible to
make products which are totally 'natural', plant-based and
preservative-free, but they would have to be safe as well as
ethical, and supplies of the natural material would have to be
regular and reliable. They would also have to perform well and
appeal to the consumer. On top of that their production would
have to be cost-effective. To be safe, they would also have to
be used within two days of purchase – and one would need a
second mortgage to pay for them. This would be fine for the
manufacturer because he wouldn't lose out, but not very good
news to the consumer. Fortunately, most consumers are not so
batty as to pay extortionate sums for a dubious privilege,
especially if a cheaper version is every bit as good.

The swing in the 1970s towards healthier living spawned a
breed of companies cashing in on the 'natural is cool'
cosmetic scene, and falsely labelling their products as
'entirely of natural origin'. As there are no legal definitions of
the word 'natural' as applied to fragrance and cosmetics in
the UK, socking 'natural' to unwary consumers is a sort of
poetic licence, applied to vulgar commerce. The consumer is
led to believe that natural is not only nicer, more pure and
better for you, but also kinder to the environment. It is
exasperating to read a label describing a product as 'natural'

merely because it has a teeny bit of herbal extract among its predominantly synthetic ingredients. A point often neglected is that just because a material is natural, it does not necessarily mean it is safe. Overall, natural materials can be more dangerous than so-called chemicals, mainly because there are far more of them and they come in many forms. Plant materials, if not monitored during preparation, can cause problems ranging from the stability of the product affecting the odour and the colour, right through to the effectiveness. On the other hand, synthetic materials can produce a superb and stable product.

A flick through a gardening book will reveal a variety of 'naturals' that are listed as 'poisonous' or that warn 'keep away from children'. These include deadly nightshade, aconite, poinsettia, foxglove and tiger lily. One of the most toxic substances known is ricin, and it is natural, occurring in the castor bean *(Ricinus communis)*. If you are still not convinced, amble on down to the library and pick up an Agatha Christie. The murder game owes much of its questionable art to natural curare, poison ivy, belladonna, cyanide and more!

However, it must be admitted that these unfriendly materials can be used to great advantage if processed correctly. Many of the plants have excellent properties – foxglove (*Digitalis purpurea*) being one of them. It yields the life-saving drug digitalis. Dried foxglove leaves are used medicinally for heart conditions. In other plants, complex materials are known to moisturise, rebuild elastin, keep the skin healthy and (one hopes) prolong its youthful look.

Most of us find it distasteful to use animal ingredients obtained by the death of an animal which has been killed for no other purpose. These ingredients are still used by a very small number of perfume manufacturers, yet there are synthetic alternatives. Where obtaining an animal-derived product causes no harm to the animal, such as lanolin, obtained from sheep wool, there is every reason to benefit from this useful material. When ingredients are procured from the bovine carcasses of creatures killed for food and leather, this may be seen as simply utilising the waste product. These waste materials can be changed into proteins, collagens and so on, which are often used successfully in skin care cosmetics. (Vegetable material can be processed into alternative types of collagen, proteins and many moisturising factors similar to those in our skin. Maybe this is where the expression 'turnip head' comes from.)

To sum up: synthetics are no more necessarily bad than naturals are necessarily good. If a plant or animal product would derive from a protected or prohibitively expensive source then, again, a synthetic or nature-identical is surely the answer.

Part of Maurene's work today is to give lectures and presentations on skin care ingredients and products. She writes: *I try to make these lectures informative, interesting to potential converts, and sometimes a dash of humour helps because science can be pretty dull stuff. Only on one occasion did I clash swords with someone. As I began to talk, after being introduced by the chairman to a particularly pleasant group of women, a florid harridan sitting in the front row rose, like Nessie from her Loch, and bellowed: 'I, for one, will not stay for one moment if you are going to talk about any skin or hair ingredients which are not natural.' Taken aback but of stoic stock, my response was: 'Dear lady, horse manure is natural. Would you put it on your skin?'*

6

ADVERSE REACTION TO COSMETICS

While millions of people worldwide use cosmetics daily without a problem, a significant number do react badly to what are normally harmless cosmetic ingredients. The most common allergens in skin care products are preservatives and perfumes. The adverse reactions suffered can come from an irritant, from an allergen, or from a combination of both. Surfactants can be irritating to the skin but have minimal allergenic properties. Some preservatives may be irritating; others may be allergenic. Any fragrance materials – plant and animal extracts or synthetic chemicals – can have irritating or allergenic properties. Adverse reactions can occur in some people after using any type of skin care product, as well as after exposure to airborne cosmetics such as hair sprays, perfumes and anti-perspirants, or even from coming into contact with other people who have used such products. Eyes and lips are particularly vulnerable areas.

Skin reactions are defined below.

Irritation
Irritation is the most common reaction in sensitive people. It is caused by a substance, often chemical, described as an irritant which can cause simple to severe problems in skin tissue.

Primary irritation is initiated by the skin being exposed to certain chemicals such as acids and alkalis which can lead to the destruction of the epidermis. The level of damage is determined by the concentration of the chemical substance and the length of time it is in contact with the skin.

Secondary irritation is caused by chemical substances which are not so damaging, for example, certain types of detergent. The skin symptoms are similar but the deleterious effects on the tissue, due to the lower chemical concentration, will produce a slower rate of damage. The reactions to irritation are localised and do not involve the immune system.

Irritant reactions are inflammation, pain, stinging and urticaria (see Glossary).

Systemic Allergic Reaction

This unusual reaction has been known to occur after exposure to a sensitizing substance by mouth, by a skin contact or by inhalation. After the sensitization, any further exposure of any part of the body to the same substance can often bring about a response from the immune system. This reaction takes place in two phases: the first is usually clinically silent, where sensitization (induction) to the allergen occurs but no reaction is noted. The second phase (elicitation) occurs when more of the same cosmetic is applied and the skin reacts within 24-48 hours by producing noticeable symptoms – a red rash, say, or swelling and intense itching which may spread over the entire body. Blisters may form and break open. More often the allergic reaction does not develop for many years – only after many repeated low-level exposures does sensitivity develop.

Unsensitized people may suffer a skin reaction if exposed to 1 per cent solution of a substance. Once sensitized, they may react to as little as a 0.001 per cent solution of the same substance. They have become hypersensitive.

Allergy to a cosmetic is diagnosed, generally by dermatologists, using a patch test. Allergens are applied to a healthy area of a patient's skin, at concentrations which should give no reaction. Any reaction suggests that the patient is allergic to that product. However, patch testing itself can cause sensitization and subsequent allergic reaction so it is important to patch test only when it is clinically necessary.

Sensitization

Sensitization means alteration of the responsiveness of the body by the presence of foreign substances (i.e. antigens) and involves the immune system. Antigens are usually proteins, although simple substances, even metals, may become antigenic by combining with and modifying the body's own proteins, which are called haptens.

Sensitization occurs when a normally safe chemical substance, for example a fragrance component, is applied to the skin and antibodies are produced. If, at some later date, the same chemical is applied, the immune system recognises it as an antigen which has previously produced antibodies in the blood, the result being an antigen antibody complex.

Photosensitization

Photosensitization is sensitization that involves the presence of light and sensitizing chemicals. The sensitizing reactions can occur with a single application of a photosensitizing substance.

Phototoxic Irritation

This skin condition develops when a chemical substance applied to the skin interacts with sunlight or ultra violet light (as used with sunbeds) causing an irritant skin reaction which may range from increased melanin production to deep, red, weeping burns.

Contamination

Anyone keen to 'try before they buy' must be aware of the possibility of picking up a viral infection from cosmetic testers found in some stores. Conjunctivitis and herpes simplex, for instance, are easily transmitted on eye make-up products and lipsticks. Sadly, even in the most prestigious of stores, cosmetic salespeople are not always correctly advised. Once when trying out a lipstick, Maurene was told discreetly by one such salesperson that she ought not to use the mascara tester as 'It could cause cystitis'. We've heard of long lashes but really!

7

PERFUMES

The word 'perfume' comes from the Latin *per* (through) and *fumus* (smoke). The earliest known perfumes were incense, used for religious purposes. Perfumes are combinations of fragrant ingredients mixed in a balanced ratio. One perfume can contain as many as 200 ingredients, so the blending – an exceedingly difficult technique carried out by a skilled perfumer – is of paramount importance to perfume manufacturers. The individual aromas are created principally to give pleasure and to attract one person to another. Equal care is taken when incorporating these perfumes into skin care products. Perfumery is usually excluded from the field of cosmetics, although perfumes are commonly manufactured in co-ordination with cosmetics.

The sense of smell is one of the body's special senses along with those of taste, vision, hearing and equilibrium. Smell and taste are both chemical senses, which means that the sensation arises from the interaction of molecules with smell or taste receptors. The art of smelling (and not stinking because one doesn't bath or shower) is called olfaction, while the sense of smell is known as the olfactory sense. Millions of receptors lie in the mucus-covered olfactory epithelium (less than one square inch in size) in the frontal part of the brain. This mucus moistens the olfactory epithelium surface and dissolves odorant gases. When we breathe in through the nostrils or mouth the air is warmed and humidified in the nasal cavity. Trigeminal nerves react to irritating odours such as pepper or ammonia with a prickling sensation, which results in sneezing. On either side of the nose, bundles of olfactory receptors extend upwards and are known collectively as the olfactory nerves. They end in the brain in masses of grey matter called the olfactory bulbs, where conscious awareness of smell begins. Electro-chemical messages are forwarded to the limbic system (the part of the brain concerned with basic emotion, sex and hunger) and the hypothalamus (a control centre in the brain concerned with thirst, hunger, satiety and other autonomic nervous system functions – see Glossary). This messaging system allows emotional and memory evoked responses to occur, so that wafts of a particular flower may remind one of one's childhood or of a particular person. People can even feel sexual excitement when smelling a particular perfume – it could be that the perfume alone evokes this feeling or because the perfume was once worn by someone desirable. The part of the brain involved with intellect (the cerebrum) also receives odour messages, which helps stimulate conscious thought and reaction.

When the hypothalamus is activated by an odour, the message goes out to all areas of the body: the endocrine (hormonal) and autonomic nervous system, and the pituitary gland (this releases into the blood-stream hormones that regulate body functions, including those that control sex, appetite and body temperature).

The inability to smell is known as anosmia. Anosmia can occur after a head injury or some damage to the odour-identifying area of the brain.

The olfactory system can warn us of impending danger – for example, by processing the odour of a burning material, it can signal to the brain the threat of fire. Insects are attracted to plants by their odours, so cross-pollination is less likely to occur. Although plant colour attracts many species, odours play a more important role. In the animal kingdom, smell is used to mark out territory as well as to send and receive information.

Pheromones are chemical substances secreted externally by
most animals, including humans. We humans all have our
very own individual natural odour. These subtle odours can
elicit a specific response from other individuals. Although
humans are not directly aware of pheromones, animals are –
their sense of smell is much keener than ours, which is why
they have no difficulty in differentiating between one human
and another. Pheromones are said to be the cause of that
seemingly irrational lust experienced for another person when
there is absolutely nothing else in common, apart from this
old primeval urge. What a shame pheromones do not take into
consideration compatibility in all aspects! They also explain
why Fido drags you from tree to lamp post, utilising his
olfactory system to savour odoriferous signals, easily distin-
guishing one smell from another. If, due to your sense of
refinement, this observation holds little appeal, consider the
races that rub noses as the initial greeting. Such an act means
two human individuals smell each other in much the same
way as Fido and a passing bitch may do. The word 'kiss' in
many languages relates to the word 'smell', and in the
western world a kiss has taken over from this rubbing of
noses.

Sense of smell is often a source of amazement and
amusement – not to mention disgust, at times. The painter
Stanley Spencer is said to have found inspiration from
sniffing around the seamier parts of a lavatory. (You could
say he was painting at his own convenience.) Yet another,
Salvador Dali, is said to have dressed his moustache with
goats' manure. As he was reputedly renowned for his
successful dalliance with ladies, the chosen dressing gives
one much to ponder.

Primitive people have always adorned the body with
odoriferous concoctions, way before the advent of what we
call perfume. Ylang Ylang flowers were spread on the bed
of newly wed Indonesian couples and the Samoans wore
garments containing these plants. Swahili women draped
jasmine flowers around the body when they wanted to
attract a member of the opposite sex. Women today use the

same principle but now the magic ingredients are usually in a tiny glass bottle. Perfume placed directly onto skin leads to interactions between its own chemical constituents and those contained in the skin itself. Some produce allergic responses, and varying reactions when exposed to sunlight. To meet this problem, perfume manufacturers have set up a system that monitors and draws up guidelines on the production of safe perfumes. The Research Institute for Fragrance Materials carries out scientific research. The results of this research are sent to the International Fragrance Association. This body recommends, restricts or suggests bans on particular substances used in the perfume industry. Although these bodies do not lay down legally binding rules, they enable manufacturers worldwide to keep within safe levels. Perfume ingredients – natural or synthetic – are one of the most common sources of allergens in cosmetic products, which is why hypo-allergic products are generally fragrance free.

Perfume Ingredients
Among the many ingredients used to make up a perfume are essential oils from plants, extracts from specific animals, alcohol, water, isolates (this is a term usually used to describe a single constituent of a volatile oil) and synthetic aromatic chemicals. Essential oils are volatile, aromatic substances found in a wide range of plants. They are extracted from a great many species of flowers, leaves, fruits, seeds, rhizomes, roots, resins, petals and barks by solvent extraction, steam distillation, mechanical pressing, maceration and enfleurage. Essential oils are added to cosmetics for their scent, for their natural 'green' marketing appeal and their supposed therapeutic effects.

Animal-derived substances were incorporated into many long-lasting fragrances, but most of these substances have now been synthetically copied and are used very minimally in modern cosmetics, due to the outrage associated with them and the expense in procuring them. Animal extracts include castoreum (castor), which is a rather

unpleasant-smelling oily secretion obtained from between
the anus and genitalia (perineal glands) of both the male
and female beaver. Ambergris is a waxy substance that
comes from secretions in the intestinal tract of the sperm
whale. Skatole is a potent-smelling, yellowish, fatty secretion that comes from the perineal glands of the civet, a
spotted cat-like mammal of Africa and south Asia. Skatole
is used as an aromatic chemical that, fortunately, in the
skilled hands of aroma scientists, can be made to produce
delightful fragrance effects in perfumes of a floral nature.
Now put your mind to this: skatole and indole are the chief
volatile constituents of the faeces being formed by the
action of the intestinal bacteria on tryptophan (an essential
amino acid). It makes you think long and hard about the
human perception of fragrance! It's hard to believe, but in
highly dilute concentration indole has a pleasant sweet
smell.

Musk – the oily, strong-smelling substance taken from
the sexual glands of the male musk deer of central Asia –
was once used in perfumes for the sole purpose of attempting to attract the opposite sex. The active constituent of
musk, muscone, is now made synthetically but there is no
duplication of natural musk. Musk ambrette was a synthetic
fixative now prohibited as a perfume ingredient due to its
potential to cause contact dermatitis and photosensitivity.
Tinctures of ambergris, castoreum, skatole and musk have
been used as fixatives in the manufacture of perfumes. (A
fixative is a substance that has the capacity to prolong
the effects of the main fragrance aroma.) Most have now
been produced synthetically (being considerably cheaper
that way) but some are still used in especially fine
fragrances. Substitutes for castoreum and skatole have been
found.

A perfume formulated from essential plant oils or animal
extracts is extremely costly. It is therefore more cost-
effective to use a combination of plant oils and synthetic
aromatic chemicals. The blend of aromatic ingredients that
forms the nucleus of a perfume is called a 'perfume

compound'. The compound is mixed with a suitable alcohol to which a percentage of water may be added, then chilled at −10°C, after which a crystal-clear product should emerge.

8

A-Z OF COMMON
INGREDIENTS

We should point out that the English spelling of ingredients is used throughout (e.g. sulphate as opposed to sulfate; aluminium instead of aluminum), although either spelling is acceptable. In brackets, following the capitalised INCI name, may be the common name, or another name by which the ingredient is popularly known.

ACACIA SENEGAL EXTRACT is obtained from the flowers and stems of the *Acacia senegal* tree that is now grown in the Middle East, USA and India. It is used in cosmetics as a thickening agent.

ACACIA SENEGAL GUM EXTRACT is derived from the gum of the *Acacia senegal* tree. This gummy extract has been used traditionally for centuries for its soothing, anti-inflammatory properties. Today's cosmetic formulators use it in dry and sensitive skin products and for thickening.

ACEROLA. (See **MALPIGHIA PUNICIFOLIA**.)

ACHILLEA MILLEFOLIUM (yarrow). A perennial herb used in astringents, hair care products, lotions, bath preparations and sun care products. It is an age-old herbal medicine used worldwide for many varied complaints, including skin diseases, ulcers, greasy skin and for stopping bleeding.

ACRYLATES COPOLYMERS are synthetic polymers. They are binders and suspending materials.

ACTINIDIA CHINENSIS (kiwi seed oil) is extracted from the seeds of the *Actinidia chinensis* (commonly known as kiwi fruit) plant. This pale yellow, light viscosity oil is very rich in C:18 acids (these can be oleic acid, linoleic acid and others). The kiwi fruit seed is used in body oils and skin care formulations for improving the condition of the skin.

ADEPS BOVIS. (See **TALLOW**.)

ALANINE is an amino acid used as a skin conditioning agent.

ALBUMEN (technically known as egg albumin or dried egg white). What is used in cosmetic manufacture is the dried egg white obtained from the eggs of chickens. It is used as a skin conditioning material.

ALCOHOL (ethanol). Pure alcohol is always a clear liquid. It is derived, in the main, by fermentation, although it can be manufactured from petrol chemicals. It is not often available naturally, apart from the fermentation of sugary juices from plants via their yeast. *(Be careful not to over-indulge in fermented fruit. You could find your bodily juices in demand by the local brewery.)* The main alcohol used is described as ethanol and comes in different strengths. Ethanol is used in some astringents, toners, aftershaves, perfumes, colognes, creams and gels. Another less frequently used alcohol is isopropanol.

ALCOHOL DENAT (denatured alcohol) is widely used in cosmetics and fragrances. It is alcohol that has been made undrinkable by the addition of a disgusting tasting substance, not only to deter the chemist from slurping instead of manufacturing or formulating with it, but to avoid the duty on it and for safety reasons (e.g. children getting hold of products containing it). In cosmetics it is an anti-foaming agent, astringent, solvent and viscosity decreasing agent.

ALEURITES MOLUCCANA (Kukui nut oil). This is obtained from the seeds of the candlenut tree, which is native to Hawaii and south-east Asia. This oil is known as *kemiri* oil in Indonesia and *lumbang* oil in the Philippines. The cold-pressed and filtered oil is clear, pale yellow and non-greasy, and although generally used to make candles and soap it is now used in moisturising lotions and sun care products. The oil is most soothing to sunburned skin as it is rapidly absorbed. Native people have used kukui oil for centuries for common skin diseases, chapped and dry skin, acne and for treating superficial burns.

ALEURITIC ACID is an organic compound that comes from shellac, a yellowish resin secreted by the *Laccifer* (*Tachardia*) *lacca* insect (see **SHELLAC**). It is used for its skin conditioning properties and is often added to perfumes.

ALGAE. Many and varied species of algae are used by cosmetic formulators, mostly for their moisturising properties. **Algae** is the EU-labelling name given to extracts from these many different species of plants.

ALGIN is the sodium salt of alginic acid which is extracted from varieties of brown seaweeds (*Phaeophyceae*). Among the brown seaweed species that are grown specifically for algin are *Alaria*, *Fucus* and *Sargassum*. Algin is used in cosmetics as a thickener, gelling agent and stabiliser.

ALKYL. Any one of a series of saturated hydrocarbons starting with methane. A product is rendered more fat soluble with one or more alkyls present.

ALLANTOIN. Extracted from the comfrey herb, allantoin is said to help regenerate and soothe damaged skin. Allantoin is also made synthetically and is used in aftershave lotions and anti-inflammatory creams for its properties that heal skin wounds and soreness.

ALMOND OIL. (See **PRUNUS AMYGDALUS AMARA** and **PRUNUS DULCIS**.)

ALOE. Extracts of many of these plants with fleshy, spiny toothed leaves of the genus *Aloe* have been used traditionally for their antibiotic, anti-inflammatory and wound healing effects. The genus *Aloe* comprises about 360 species which are chiefly native to Africa, but are now distributed throughout the dry regions of the world. (Although saying that, many are of course raised as houseplants in countries at sub-zero temperatures!) *Aloe vera* is one of the species to have achieved particular popularity in cosmetic use recently. *Aloe vera* is the name for the species also known as *Aloe barbadensis,* which is the official INCI name for extracts of this plant.

ALOE BARBADENSIS. This is the EU-labelling name for extracts and derivatives of the lily-like aloe plant native to South Africa, the *Aloe barbadensis*. (The classification of this plant seems to vary: sometimes it is said to belong to the aloe family, at other times it is said to belong to the lily family.) Aloe barbadensis extract is taken from the leaves of the plant, which possess the remarkable ability to close their pores completely, thereby avoiding water loss. The centre of each leaf is filled with a clear gel and it is this that has superb healing properties, particularly good for burns. The gel consists of about 98 per cent water, plus vitamins, minerals, enzymes, glycoproteins, aloins, albumen, anthraquinones, silica and amino acids, plus many other components. Aloe barbadensis flower extract is derived from the flowers of this aloe; aloe barbadensis gel is the actual juice that is expressed from the leaves. The gel is used as a humectant and for its skin softening properties in skin creams today, just as it was in ancient Egypt some three thousand years ago. The Romans, in particular, grew it and used it for healing wounds.

ALPHA-HYDROXY ACIDS (commonly known as **AHAs**) are natural acids derived from fruit, milk and sugar cane, and which have exfoliating and emollient properties. These acids include glycolic acid (from sugar cane), pyruvic acid (from papaya), lactic acid (from milk), malic acid (from apples), tartaric acid (from wine) and citric acid (from citrus fruits). They help the skin to shed dead cells. These ingredients are common in mature skin products because of this and because of the AHAs' ability, under certain circumstances, to be moisturising and hydrating. In products for ageing skins, the acids are designed to 'peel' the skin, giving it a more youthful appearance by smoothing very fine wrinkles. On young skins the products promote the advantages of ridding the superficial skin layers of comedones (blackheads) and an oily appearance. AHAs are often produced synthetically too.

ALUM (see **POTASSIUM ALUM**). Alum is a whitish mineral salt, chemically referred to as a double sulphate of aluminium sulphate and potassium sulphate. It is used in many industries including the cosmetics industry, where it is used in astringent formulations. It is extracted from earth or rock in some parts of the world. Alum has been used in Britain for centuries for material dyeing, papermaking, tanning and medicinal purposes.

ALUMINIUM ACETATE. (See **ALUMINIUM SALTS**.)

ALUMINIUM CHLORIDE. (See **ALUMINIUM SALTS**.)

ALUMINIUM CHLOROHYDRATE. (See **ALUMINIUM SALTS**.)

ALUMINIUM HYDROXIDE – an inorganic compound used in cosmetics as an opacifying agent.

ALUMINIUM PHENOSULPHONATE. (See **ALUMINIUM SALTS**.)

ALUMINIUM POTASSIUM SULPHATE is a technical name for alum. (See **POTASSIUM ALUM**.)

ALUMINIUM SALTS. There are many of these acid salts of aluminium such as aluminium acetate, phenosulphonate, chloride, hydroxide, chlorohydrate and many more, although aluminium chlorohydrate is the only one in common use. Aluminium salts are used mainly to prevent sweating (to a degree) and to prevent body odour caused by bacteria breaking down. They do so by blocking sweat from reaching the skin. Aluminium chloride was the first and most effective salt used for commercial products but is now seldom used. While antiseptic, it has been known to cause skin irritation and allergic reaction in some people, so the safer aluminium chlorohydrate is more commonly used.

ALUMINIUM STARCH OCTENYLSUCCINATE – an aluminium salt used as an anti-caking agent and as an absorbent.

ALUMINIUM STEARATE – a cosmetic colouring additive. This is the aluminium salt of stearic acid. (It is white but imparts colour when in solution.)

ALUMINIUM ZIRCONIUM TETRACHLOROHY-DREX GLY is an amino acid derivative and inorganic salt, used in astringents and deodorants.

AMBERGRIS is a waxy substance that comes from secretions in the intestinal tract of the sperm whale. Years ago it was widely used as a fixative in perfumes, but now synthetic substitutes are more commonly used.

AMINO ACIDS are the basic structure from which proteins are made. Most can be produced by the body but some come solely from food sources. Amino acids repair damaged muscle tissue and build new connective tissue and are therefore very necessary to healthy skin. They are added to emollients and moisturisers because of their ability to be absorbed by the skin. Collagen amino acids come from the protein-rich white fibres of animal connective tissue, cartilage and bone, which are changed into gelatin by heating. Cosmetic manufacturers in some cases have discreetly dropped the name 'animal'. The same applies in the case of elastin amino acids and keratin amino acids. Elastin is a protein derived from connective tissue, and keratin is taken from animal hairs, hooves, horns and feathers. Increasingly plant-derived alternatives are being developed. They are not always identical chemically but similar, and with similar properties in finished products.

AMNIOTIC FLUID is the fluid found within the amniotic sac of pregnant cows between three to six months' gestation. It is a sterile yellow liquid of pH7, and is used in facial and body moisturising products.

ANACARDIUM OCCIDENTALE. (Cashew nut oil.) The oil is extracted from the seeds of the South American tree *Anacardium occidentale*, native to the north east coastal area of Brazil. Generally known as the cashew tree, it produces a fleshy receptacle, commonly called an apple, at the end of which is the well-known kidney shaped nut. The whole tree is utilised for a wide range of products. Native Americans and Africans used the bark for malarial fevers, and the fresh shell juice was good for removing warts and corns. A gum with the same qualities as gum Arabic is found in the cashew plant.

This is imported from South America under the name Acaju gum, which is used by local bookbinders that wash their books with it to keep away moths and ants. The caustic oil found in the layers of the fruit has been rubbed into the floors of Indian houses to keep white ants at bay. It is used in cosmetics for its skin conditioning properties.

ANNATTO is the red pigment that is derived from the seeds of the tropical *Bixa orellana* tree. The EU-labelling name for annatto is CI 75120. Special regulations regarding the use of this substance are required by cosmetic formulators. (See also **BIXA ORELLANA**.)

ANTHEMIS NOBILIS (chamomile). This is the EU-labelling name given to the extract and oil derived from the flowers of the true chamomile plant *Chamaemelum nobile*, synonym *Anthemis nobilis*. It is also known as Roman, common or English chamomile. There are other members of the chamomile family that are also used in cosmetics (see **CHAMOMILEA RECUTITA**). Several of the natural chemicals in these chamomile oils have properties which contribute to their ancient reputation for wound healing. The oil has a potent sedative and anti-inflammatory effect which is believed to help skin that has been damaged by overexposure to the sun or where the skin's natural defences have been reduced by exposure to detergents such as those used when washing up.

ANTIOXIDANTS are ingredients that help to prevent spoilage when certain substances come into contact with oxygen. Oxygen is a powerful element that can spoil fats and oils and give them an offensive rancid smell. Vitamin E (or tocopherol), beta carotene and Vitamin C are commonly known antioxidants. BHT (butylated hydroxy toluene) is another. Antioxidant also applies to the ingredient capabilities in counteracting free radical effects in products, which are said to slow down the ageing process. Skin care cosmetics that contain antioxidants such as Vitamins E and C, tocopherols, beta-carotene and flavonoids (anti free radical compounds found in plants) counter free radical damage done to the skin by decomposing the free radicals into

certain components which a healthy body is able to fight
off. Many of these antioxidants which inactivate free radicals are found in nuts, fruit and vegetables, hence the
importance of having a balanced diet. Antioxidants living in
the skin can be destroyed by the UV radiation of sunlight,
leaving a path open to attack from free radicals. The greater
the damage, the lower the antioxidant levels fall, resulting
in damage to the collagen, elastin, cell membranes and
nuclear constituents within the skin, causing skin cancer and
wrinkling. While it is beneficial to build up the body with
antioxidant supplements, it is doubtful that the skin will get
any protection from them as the body will use them up
before the skin is reached. That is why cosmetic companies
are manufacturing cosmetics containing antioxidants, which
can be applied directly to the skin where they can fight free
radicals instantly. Clinical tests by dermatologists in the
USA say these antioxidants need to penetrate through the
stratum corneum to be useful. They need to contain concentrations of between 2 and 10 per cent in a product to be
effective. They conclude that destroying excessive free
radicals by using antioxidants in cosmetics offers a chance
for slowing down the ageing process by preventing the
formation of new wrinkles. However, if you have wrinkles
already, antioxidants in cosmetics are not going to do much
at all.

ANTISEPTICS. These ingredients are included in certain
products to help reduce the risk of infections from micro-
organisms. The balance of micro-organisms on the skin can
easily be upset, during stressful periods, when one is ill,
careless with hygiene or even over-zealous with it. Scouring
the skin with strong substances can remove both the good and
bad 'creepies'. Two of the many antiseptics are triclosan and
cetrimide. A powerful antiseptic that saved countless lives in
the First World War was carbolic acid.

AORTA EXTRACT is taken from the aorta, the main
artery in animals which transports blood away from the heart.
Extracts are used in creams for ageing skins.

AQUA (water) is one of the most commonly used ingredients in skin care cosmetic formulating, and the only single ingredient that can be 90 per cent of a product. Water is used as a dilutant and as a solvent and dispersing medium for other ingredients. Different types of water can have different effects – trace metal ions could be present in water from a particular source so causing discolouring and other detrimental effects to the product. High quantities of magnesium and calcium salts produce lime soaps that affect emulsification. Microbes may even contaminate water. However, if a pure water is used (and that differs from purified mountain water, de-ionised water and herbal waters), problems like these are generally avoided. Pure water rarely occurs in nature because of its capacity to dissolve varying substances in large amounts. The hardness of natural water is caused mainly by the presence of calcium and magnesium salts, and to a lesser degree by other metals including aluminium and iron. Some of the hardness of water can be removed by boiling, sterilizing it at the same time.

ARACHIDIC ACID is a fatty acid occurring as glycerides in peanut and other vegetable oils. It is a cleansing and opacifying material. Its technical name is Eicosanoic Acid.

ARACHIDONIC ACID is a skin conditioning material. It is an essential fatty acid present in the skin as well as in the liver, brain, glands and fat of humans and animals. It is the principal fatty acid of the adrenal gland. The acid is generally derived from animal liver for use in cosmetics, predominantly for its emollient, skin smoothing and healing properties. It is found particularly in skin lotions for soothing eczema and rashes.

ARACHIDYL BEHENATE – an ester used as a skin conditioning agent.

ARACHIS HYPOGAEA (peanut, groundnut or monkey nut). Seeds of the peanut plant *Arachis hypogaea* are crushed to exude the oil that is used in soaps, baby products, emollients and night creams. It is often used in cosmetic preparations as a substitute for almond and olive oil. Peanut flour is also used in cosmetics, and is obtained by grinding the peanuts.

ARGANIA SPINOSA OIL is a fixed oil obtained from

the expressed kernels of the African tree known as *Argania spinosa*. It is a skin conditioning material and is used in cosmetics for its emollient and occlusive properties.

ARNICA MONTANA (arnica). This extract derives from the dried flower heads of the perennial alpine herb *Arnica montana*, also known as wolf's bane. It has been used medicinally for hundreds of years for sore throats, for combating fever and for improving circulation and relieving congestion. Externally it is good for bruises, sprains and acne. It is used only occasionally and at very low levels in cosmetics due to its toxicity.

ARROWROOT EXTRACT. (See **MARANTA ARUNDINACEA**.)

ASCORBIC ACID (a technical name of Vitamin C) is an organic compound and is used as an antioxidant and pH adjuster in skin creams (see **VITAMINS**).

ASCORBYL PALMITATE is an antioxidant. It is an ester of ascorbic acid and palmitic acid.

AVENA SATIVA (oat extract). Oat is a well-known cereal grain found on many a breakfast table. Not so well known, perhaps, is its use in cosmetics, particularly those designed for skins irritated by conditions such as psoriasis or allergic dermatitis. Oat contains a colloid that has a soothing effect on skin, particularly that which is sensitive and/or sunburned. It also makes the skin feel smooth and provides the product with viscosity and emulsion stability.

AZULENE. The azulene used for cosmetic purposes applies to the blue oils that result when essential oils from many plants are distilled or heated. Generally, this hydrocarbon is extracted from the chamomile plant or produced synthetically. It is used in cosmetics as a skin conditioning material. In chemistry terms, azulene is also a blue crystalline solid, an aromatic compound converted to naphthalene on heating.

BAOBAB SEED OIL (it is also known as the Cream of Tartar tree, and Mbuyu in Swahili) is extracted from the gourd-like fruit of the baobab tree *Adansonia digitata*, which can live for thousands of years. The edible pulp contains up to one hundred bean-sized seeds from which the oil is cold-pressed and filtered. For centuries Africans have applied baobab oil to their skins to treat disorders such as psoriasis and eczema, and to relieve sores, inflammation, fever, toothache, insect bites and it is used as a malaria prophylactic. It is also massaged into muscles to relieve aches and pains. In the pulp of the long fat pods are tartaric acid, mucilage, pectin and tartrates, hence the name 'Cream of Tartar tree'. The odd appearance of this squat tree, which appears to have been uprooted by some powerful hand and placed upside down, has resulted in many superstitious uses. Its survival ploy, however, is to be too fat to fell easily, plus the wood is light and spongy so any potential assassin's axe is more likely to bounce off the wood than cut it. A good tree may hold about one thousand gallons of water so it also makes poor firewood and charcoal. It is sometimes used as a fixed oil, and in astringents.

BARIUM SULPHATE – an inert cosmetic colouring additive that is white initially, but imparts colour when suspended in solution.

BEESWAX. (See **CERA ALBA**.)

BEESWAX (SYNTHETIC) is made from mineral oil.

BENTONITE is a colloidal aluminium silicate clay that swells as it absorbs water. In cosmetics, this absorption ability allows it to form a gelatinous mass. It is used to thicken lotions and to suspend make-up pigments, of particular use in face masques where it absorbs oil on the face and reduces shine.

BENZENECARBALDEHYDE (benzaldehyde) is a yellowish volatile oily liquid that is found in almond kernels. It smells of almond too. It is used in the manufacture of perfumes.

BENZOIC ACID is an aromatic acid that occurs naturally in cherry bark, raspberries, tea, anise and cassia bark. It is also a pH adjuster and preservative. In cosmetics its main use is to protect products against moulds and yeast.

BENZYL ALCOHOL is an aromatic alcohol component; used in cosmetics as a preservative, solvent, viscosity decreasing agent or flavouring.

BETA CAROTENE (provitamin A). This vitamin is

obtained from natural sources and is also prepared synthetically. It is well known as the natural colour in egg yolks,
butter, carrots and pumpkin. It is occasionally used in colouring cosmetics and has skin conditioning properties. It may be
better known by its technical name: B-Carotene.

BHA. This is short for butylated hydroxy anisole, a
synthetic, edible antioxidant.

BHT. This is short for butylated hydroxy toluene. It is a
synthetically made, food grade phenol derivative used as an
antioxidant.

BIOFLAVONOIDS. These flavonoid compounds are
obtained by extraction of citrus rinds. These biological
materials have antioxidant and anti-inflammatory properties.

BIOLOGICAL ADDITIVES are generally substances
derived from the glands and tissues of various species of
animals. These include amniotic fluid, keratin, collagen,
elastin, hyaluronic acid, placenta and blood derivatives. They
are added to cosmetic formulations for varied reasons (see
individual entries). The term biological additive could also
refer to plant additives, including essential oils from plants;
and petrol, mineral oil, petroleum jelly, etc. are fractions of
petroleum oil which is biological, in being derived from
animals thousands of years ago.

BIOTIN is a vitamin of the B complex. It is present in
small amounts of every living cell, and particularly abundant
in egg yolk and liver. Deficiency of biotin in humans is
considered extremely rare. It is added to some cosmetic
formulations because of this organic compound's skin conditioning properties.

BISABOLOL is an alcohol (terpene) used as a skin
conditioning agent.

BITTER ALMOND EXTRACT. (See **PRUNUS AMYG-
DALUS AMARA**.)

BIXA ORELLANA is the EU-labelling name for extracts
from the seed of *Bixa orellana*, a tree which originated in
tropical America but which is now grown in many tropical
countries. The red pigment of the waxy red seeds is made into
a paste and used by Amazonians to paint their faces. Bixa

orellana extract comes from the fleshy plant tissue, and Bixa orellana seed extract comes from the crushed seeds of the *Bixa orellana*. The red colouring, known as annatto, is obtained by washing the pulpy seeds with water. It is often used in sunscreen and after-sun products and baby care products.

BLACKCURRANT OIL. (See **RIBES NIGRUM**.)

BLOOD DERIVATIVES. Blood is extracted from cows and then treated to remove unwanted substances. A dried water-soluble yellow powder results. This is added to cosmetics, particularly creams that are supposed to rejuvenate and aftershave products, because it is generally believed that the extract stimulates the absorption of oxygen. Serum albumin (which is the major protein component of blood plasma), blood extract and fibronectin (a glycoprotein) are all used in cosmetic formulation and all originally derive from bovine blood.

BOMBYX (silk worm extract) is a material extracted from squashed silkworms, the larvae of the Chinese moth *Bombyx mori* that eats only mulberry tree leaves. (It has been so domesticated in China that it cannot fly any more. It is the very same moth that manufactures silk for us.) Silk amino acids, however, are obtained from silk by hydrolysis, and are used in moisturising preparations. Silk has been used to add bulk to cosmetics, although now there are cheaper materials. (See also **SERICA**.)

BORAGO OFFICINALIS is the EU-labelling name given to extracts of the stout annual herb, *Borage officinalis*. This herb, with its characteristic star-shaped blue flowers, is native to the Mediterranean though commonly found in central Europe, north Africa and in the waste grounds near human habitation and arable fields of many temperate areas. Borage extract comes from the herby part of the plant and is used for its skin conditioning properties. Borage seed oil is extracted from the seeds which have a high concentration of GLA (gamma linolenic acid). GLA is important for good health.

BORIC ACID is an inorganic acid and cosmetic biocide.

Boric acid is used in skin care cosmetics for its antiseptic properties, which act as a fungicide and a bacteriocide.

BRASSICA OLEIFERA (rapeseed oil) is the oil derived from the rapeseed plant, *Brassica campestris,* the turnip-like Eurasian fodder plant which is now also cultivated for its oil-bearing seeds. It is this flower that produces a wonderful blaze of yellow in arable fields in Britain. Rapeseed oil is expressed from the seeds of *Brassica campestris*. The crushed seeds produce unpleasant-smelling brownish yellow oil. It is used in soft soaps and as a lubricant.

2-BROMO-2 NITROPROPANE-1,3-DIOL. (See **PRESERVATIVES**.)

BRONOPOL. (See **PRESERVATIVES**.)

BUTTER is the general term in the cosmetic industry for any product solid at normal room temperature that melts when the temperature is increased to that of the body. Cocoa butter (*Theobroma cacao*) is one of the most commonly used in the cosmetics industry. Butter itself is the semi-solid fat containing water that is made from cows' milk, and is used as a skin conditioning agent in cosmetics.

BUTYL is the name of a certain chemical group.

BUTYL METHOXY DIBENZOYLMETHANE is a substituted aromatic compound and is considered to be a highly efficient ultra violet light absorber, so is added to some sunscreen products.

BUTYLENE GLYCOL (or butene glycol) is used in creams and lotions as a viscosity decreasing agent and solvent.

BUTYLPARABEN. (See **PRESERVATIVES**.)

BUTYROSPERMUM PARKII is the EU-labelling name given to extracts of Shea butter, a fat obtained from the nuts of the karite tree, *Butyrospermum parkii*, which grows in swamps in West and Central African countries. Shea butter is an excellent emollient, providing a good 'slip', so it is predominantly used in creams. It protects the skin from dehydration and other influences of climate. Shea butter extract derives from shea butter. The fraction of the butter that is not saponifed during the refining process is known as shea butter unsaponifiables. See Glossary.

BUXUS CHINENSIS (jojoba extract) is derived from the nuts of the small desert shrub jojoba, *Buxus chinensis.* From the seeds of the plant an oil is extracted, and from this oil a wax is derived. It is a good emollient, imparting a smooth, silky feel to the skin, and it may well help sooth acne and psoriasis. It is particularly popular for use as a natural scrub bead in scrub gels, soaps and exfoliating products.

Maurene noted that in researching the ways of a particular North American Red Indian tribe (she refuses to identify them for fear of alopecia!), she was impressed with their medicinal, culinary and beautifying uses of the jojoba plant. She says: 'However, not even 12 years air hostessing prepared me for their novel method of contraception. (I hasten to add I allude to my knowledge of the theory only.) This comprised dipping birds' feathers into the jojoba wax and then, my dear, inserting the greasy mass into one's vagina. Is there no end to the human imagination? No wonder birds fly away from humans, some squawking raucously as they flee!'

C12-15 ALCOHOLS are fatty alcohols, used as emulsion stabilisers and viscosity increasing agents.

C20-40 ALKYL STEARATE. Simply put, this is an ester of stearic acid and fatty alcohols with 20-40 carbon atoms in.

CACTUS (CEREUS GRANDIFLORUS) EXTRACT. This particular ingredient is extracted from the flowers of the cactus *Cereus grandiflorus,* a night-blooming cactus native to Mexico and tropical America. It has heady vanilla scented flowers that open in the desert's cool night air. In cosmetics it is used for its skin tightening and moisturising ability. Most members of the cacti family, like other arid region plants, survive by storing any available moisture so they can function during long dry spells. Unlike our friend the camel, they can be delightfully scented and breathtakingly coloured, yet, like those ships of the desert, they die if their water reservoir dries up. Other cacti used in cosmetic formulations include *Opuntia tuna*, commonly known as the prickly pear, which is cultivated in orchards of the United States and Mexico. The pear comprises 83 per cent water, 10 per cent sucrose with the remaining 7 per cent a composition of tartaric acid and citric acids, mucilage and other mucopolysaccharides. The inside slimy, succulent material is processed for use in moisturisers, and can be used in sunscreen products. The *Cactaceae* family, consisting of around 2,500 species, is widely used in manufacturing lip salves, balms and creams. The *Yucca* genus contains saponins and tannins, which are used in cosmetics for their foaming and astringent properties. (*Incidentally, should one be bitten by the odd tarantula while walking Fido among the sand dunes, then the pulp from the Opuntia's leaf is the answer. Made into a poultice and applied to the bite, it takes away the awful stinging, burning sensation and reduces the swelling post haste.*)

The *Lophophora williamsii* species (commonly known as peyote) from northern Mexico contains an alkaloid called mescalin, which, if eaten, produces intoxicating and hallucinogenic effects on the brain. The tubercles (called mescal buttons) of the plant are dried and then sliced and chewed. Both the Navajo and Huichol Indians are familiar with these innocent looking 'buttons'. *Echinocactus grusonii*, a large barrel shaped Mexican cactus, was historically used to quench thirst as well as to moisturise and protect skin.

Not all cacti live in arid regions – the genus *Rhipsalis* is one of several which can be found hanging from forest trees that grow in tropical America as well as in equatorial Africa, Sri Lanka and Madagascar.

CALAMINE is a substance made from zinc oxide with about 0.5 per cent ferric oxide added to it. It is inorganic, absorbent and an opacifying agent. It is used in lotions for its astringent, soothing and cooling properties. It is well known for its therapeutic effect on sunburned and chicken pox afflicted skin.

CALCIUM CARBONATE is an inorganic salt used to add bulk to a product, as a buffering agent and a pH adjuster.

CALCIUM STEARATE is a calcium salt of a fatty acid known as stearic acid.

CALENDULA OFFICINALIS OIL. The oil is obtained from the peeled flowers of the marigold *Calendula officinalis,* an annual herbaceous plant. Marigold has been used in folk medicine for centuries for skin diseases and to help alleviate menstruation pains. This infused (soaked to extract properties) oil is used to heal abrasions, and, being a particularly gentle oil, is recommended for use in baby skin care products. It is found in other cosmetics including lip balms, sunscreen products and shampoos.

CALOPHYLLUM OIL (*Calophyllum inophyllum*) is extracted from the oily seeds of the tropical Santa Maria tree. It is used in moisturising creams. Natives of Papua New Guinea, Samoa and New Caledonia utilise the leaves for skin problems; Fijians use the oil as a liniment for joint pains, arthritis, bruises and coral wounds. One of the constituents, calophyllolide, is noted for reducing histamine inflammation in rats.

CAMELINA SATIVA (Gold of Pleasure Oil) is obtained from the seeds of a cultivated plant *Camelina sativa*, which was, at one time, a common weed in cereal crops. It is used in many creams as a skin conditioning agent.

CAMELLIA KISSI OIL is extracted from the seeds of *Camellia kissi*, ornamental shrubs with glossy evergreen leaves and pink, red or white flowers. Extracts from many varieties of *Camellia* have been used in the Orient for centuries, and the plants have been used in hair care treatments in Asia for hundreds of years. A plant ingredient much revered by Japanese fair persons! Camellia kissi oil is added to skin care products for its emollient and skin conditioning properties.

CAMELLIA OLEIFERA (extract) is obtained from the leaves of *Camellia oleifera,* a tea plant. In cosmetics it acts as an anti-inflammatory and is an antioxidant.

CAMELLIA SINENSIS (oil) is derived from the leaves of another species of tea plant, *Camellia sinensis*, (known as Green Tea or China tea). The leaf of this plant is brewed to make this well-known drink. It is one of the most widely cultivated members of the genus *Camellia,* and the most important economically. In cosmetics it is found in some anti-cellulite products, and is used as a skin soother and antioxidant.

CAMPHOR OIL is a sweet-smelling essential oil extracted from the roots, branches and wood of the Oriental species of the camphor evergreen tree (*Cinnamomum camphora*). It is a by-product of camphor production and only contains small amounts of camphor. The Chinese used Borneo camphor for embalming as well as in their traditional medicine.

CANDELILLA CERA is the wax that is produced from an extraction of the plant *Euphorbia cerifera*, a species from the genus *Euphorbia*. The name 'candelilla' means little candle and 'cera' means wax. The plant may be found in Latin America, particularly Mexico. *Euphorbia cerifera* plants are found in abundance in rocky deserts. The plant's outer coating is extracted for use in various cosmetics, fragrances and liquid powders as a binder and as a viscocity increasing agent.

CANDELILLA WAX. (See **CANDELILLA CERA**.)

CANOLA OIL is a Canadian modified rapeseed oil extracted from the *Brassica napus* species. It is low in erucic acid, which is related to oleic acid but is not edible. Because canola oil is low in erucic acid yet high in oleic and other acids, it is edible. In cosmetics it is a skin conditioning agent.

CAPRYLIC/CAPRIC/LAURIC TRIGLYCERIDE is an oily mixture derived from coconut oil with good spreading ability. Basically, it is an ester of glycerine and caprylic, capric and lauric acids. It is used extensively in creams and lotions where it promotes penetration onto the skin and is non-greasy. It serves as a vehicle for dispersion of pigment in bath oils.

CARAMEL is basically the solution created when sugar or glucose is heated, along with a little alkali, or trace mineral acid added. In cosmetics it is used as a colouring agent and a skin soothing agent. This caramel differs from that a cook may produce in a kitchen by being carefully made by controlled chemical processes.

CARBOMERS are, in general, a group of substances used in cosmetic formulations to emulsify, thicken and stabilise.

When neutralised, these slightly acidic powders form thick clear gels which can thicken emulsions.

CARMINE is a crimson colour added to cosmetic products. It is derived from cochineal, a Mexican cactus-eating insect called *Coccus cacti*. The red pigment is extracted from the crushed dried female insects. (See also **COLOURS**.)

CARNAUBA WAX. (See **COPERNICIA CERIFERA**.)

CARRAGEENAN. (See **CHONDRUS CRISPUS**.)

CARTHAMUS TINCTORIUS (safflower). This oil comes from the seeds of the thistle-like Eurasian plant with orange and red flowers, *Carthamus tinctorius*, commonly known as safflower. The oil is used in skin creams for its softening properties. Some people confuse safflower with saffron, but these are actually completely different plants. Safflower extract is obtained from the flowers of this species of safflower.

CASTOR OIL. (See **RICINUS COMMUNIS**.)

CASTOREUM (castor) is an animal extract – a rather unpleasant-smelling oily secretion obtained from between the anus and genitalia (perinea glands) of both the male and female beaver. It used to be widely used as a fixative in the manufacture of perfumes (a fixative here is a substance that has the capacity of prolonging the effects of the main fragrance aroma) but synthetic substitutes are now more commonly produced. By the way, castor oil is totally unrelated to this – the nauseating vegetable oil made from the castor bean, *Ricinus communis*, was commonly used many years ago to relieve constipation.

CELLULOSE GUM – the sodium salt of cellulose used as an emulsion stabiliser.

CENTAUREA CYANUS (cornflower) is obtained from the dried flowers of the *Centaurea cyanus* cornflower. For centuries it has been used in Europe as a traditional remedy for weak eyes, and still today it is found in some skin care products designed for use around the eyes. Cornflower extract is also used to alleviate inflamed eyes, bruises, wounds and skin ulcers.

CERA ALBA (beeswax). This is an exceptionally rich

white wax obtained from the honeycomb in the hive of the bee. This is another favourite ingredient for emulsion formulae. The oldest emulsifier was probably the beeswax/borax combination used to formulate cold creams. The colour and characteristics of the wax depends very much on the area in which the wax is found, in much the same way that the location of the hive is reflected in the condition and the taste of the honey. Most of the constituents are made in the eight abdominal glands of the bee. These are mainly hydrocarbons, wax acids, wax esters and polyesters, the resultant wax being chewed by a worker bee in order to build the cells in the hives. Recent research into the chemical composition of beeswax (in particular, yellow untreated beeswax, *Cera flava*) has revealed its versatility. It keeps moisture within the skin for longer than traditional moisturisers by providing a barrier yet still maintains the skin's permeability for smaller molecules to pass through. It also does not oxidise easily due to its stable constituents, and any artificial antioxidants are reduced by the presence of natural antioxidants in the beeswax itself.

CERA MICROCRISTALLINA (microcrystalline wax) is a wax produced by processing petroleum. It has fine crystals, quite different from the bigger crystals of paraffin wax. It can be described as a long chain of saturated hydrocarbons. This wax is sometimes used as a beeswax substitute (for beeswax is a lot more expensive). It is used in skin care preparations as an emulsion stabiliser and viscosity increasing material.

CERAMIDES. It is very much in vogue to incorporate into certain products compounds which have been formulated to match those occurring naturally in the skin, in particular compounds known to diminish with age, health problems or environmental influences. A small important group called ceramides was discovered as early as the 1800s. Ceramides – natural skin components – are present in the stratum corneum (the uppermost layer in the epidermis) and their role is to structure and maintain the water retention capacity of the skin. This important discovery has led cosmetic chemists and pharmacists to match such important skin compounds. This has been accomplished using various sources such as plants, animals and yeast as well as through chemical synthesization, and ceramides are available in various products now marketed. Their role in cosmetic products is to improve skin structure and texture. Claims have also been made for their ability to normalise the water content of damaged skin.

CERESIN. This is a naturally occurring wax-like mineral which is basically a complex combination of hydrocarbons produced by the purification of ozokerite with sulphuric acid and is filtered to form hard waxy cakes. It is used in the cosmetic industry as an anti-static agent, a binder and to help form stable emulsions. It is used in protective creams as well as functioning as a thickener.

CEREUS GRANDIFLORUS. (See **CACTUS EXTRACT**.)

CETEARETH COMPOUNDS are cetearyl alcohol ethoxylates. Cetearyl alcohol is not a single substance but is the name used for various natural or synthetic blends of cetyl alcohol and stearyl alcohol. **CETEARETH 30** is a waxy solid that arises from a reaction of cetyl alcohol and 30 molecules of ethylene oxide. Cetearth 30 (and other numbers) is used in cosmetics as an emollient, emulsifer, antifoam agent and lubricant.

CETEARYL ALCOHOL comes from animal or vegetable sources and is a mixture of fatty alcohols, mainly cetyl and stearyl, and helps in the manufacture of smooth emulsions.

CETEARYL OCTANOATE is used in skin conditioning creams and lotions and is noted for its efficient water-repelling capabilities. Derived from either palm kernel or coconut, as well as being a synthetic ester, cetearyl octanoate corresponds to the preen gland oil of water-fowl. It protects the skin from drying out.

CETETH 20 – an emulsifier reactive with oil-in-water creams and lotions. Generally a ceteth is a compound of derivatives of cetyl, lauryl, stearyl and oleyl alcohols reacted with 20 molecules of ethylene oxide.

CETOSTEARYL ALCOHOL is a blend of cetyl alcohol and stearyl alcohol, which are derived from stearic acid or palmitic acid from tallow or palm oil. It is an emulsifying and stabilising wax produced from the reduction of these plant oils and natural waxes. It is also used as an emollient and to give a product viscosity.

CETYL ACETATE – the ester of cetyl alcohol and acetic acid. It is used as a skin conditioning agent and as a moisturiser.

CETYL ALCOHOL is a fatty alcohol, a waxy crystalline and solid substance found in spermaceti or palm oil. It is also found in coconut and other vegetable oils, as well as being made synthetically. It is used extensively to stabilise emulsions, as a viscosity increasing agent and as an emulsifying agent in many cosmetic preparations. Its toxicity level on skin is low and is considered to be non-comedogenic.

CETYL ESTERS (technically known as synthetic spermaceti wax) are a blend of esters, primarily of the cetyl alcohol esters with lauric acid, palmitic acid, myristic acid and stearic acid. Used in cosmetics as a stabiliser, thickener and to give body and opacity to skin care creams, they impart a soft feel to the skin. Cetyl esters are used to replace, and are virtually indistinguishable from, natural spermaceti wax which used to be obtained from the head of the sperm whale. The latter source of spermaceti is no longer used in cosmetic manufacture.

CETYL PALMITATE (also once known as synthetic spermaceti) is an ester with the same chemical properties and structure of whale spermaceti. It is produced by the reaction of cetyl alcohol and palmitic acid. It thickens and stabilises emulsions, and is used as a skin conditioner.

CETYL PHOSPHATE is a phosphorus compound, used as a surfactant and emulsifying agent.

CETYL RICINOLEATE is the cetyl ester of castor oil acids used in tanning preparations. It is an emollient and emulsion stabiliser.

CHAMOMILE. (See **ANTHEMIS NOBILIS**.)

CHAMOMILLA RECUTITA (of the species *Matricaria recutita*, also known as Matricaria chamomilla) is the annual soothingly aromatic herb which is commonly known as wild chamomile, German or Hungarian chamomile. Chamomilla recutita is the EU-labelling name given to the extract and the oil which derives from the German chamomile herb, *Chamomilla recutita*. The flowers, with some leaves, are steam distilled to produce the oil. This plant is found in most of Europe and has been widely used for centuries for digestive disorders, sore throats and catarrh. Chamomile is perhaps most well known for its use in making chamomile tea. In cosmetics, it is used for its antiseptic and anti-inflammatory properties, in compresses and bath preparations.

CHIA OIL. (See **SALVIA HISPANICA**.)

CHINESE HERBS have been used by Oriental civilisations for centuries for their therapeutic qualities, and some are now incorporated into modern skin care products, in particular sun care preparations and bath products. Plant extracts such as the vegetable *Hui Xian* are generally rich in mineral salts and mucins (glycoproteins – substances in plants that cement cells together), which regulate the moisture content of the skin, and also contain elements that form a thin film over the skin. Others including *Po Zhulin Hua* (Water Nymph Lotus) and *Tung Kua* (Oriental Giant Gourd) are used in sun care preparations. Japanese formulators have incorporated herbs such as *Ling Ling Xiang* (Oriental lovage) and *Maoxiang* (geranium grass) into bath preparations predominantly for their soothing effects. *Hua Gua* (Oriental cucumber) is used in skin care preparations for its many properties including (it is said) the ability temporarily to reduce the appearance of facial wrinkles, achieved by its amino acids action, which tightens the skin. Another herb, *Wu Tung* (the Moon-Cake Seeds tree or the Japanese Cosmetic Tung tree) is used in many and varied skin creams, as is *Long Xu Cai* (Dragon's Tongue).

CHITIN. A white powder, it is a component of the shells of crustaceans, insects, arachnids and centipedes and some fungi. Chitin used in cosmetics is derived from the protective structure of marine animals that do not have a backbone. It is used as an abrasive. **Chitosan**, which is deacetylated chitin, is used in wound healing emulsions, tanning and hair care products.

CHLOROPHYLL, the green pigment of plants, contains healing and soothing properties. It is also used as a natural colouring agent. It has a mild deodorising effect, so is included in many antiperspirants, deodorants and mouthwashes.

CHLOROXYLENOL – a cosmetic biocide and used in deodorants as a preservative.

CHOLESTEROL is a fatty substance found in plant and animal tissues, blood, bile and animal fats. It can be used in cosmetics as a skin conditioning agent, moisturiser, emulsifier and lubricant.

CHONDRUS CRISPUS (carrageenan) is the plant matter that is extracted from varieties of the red seaweed, *Rhodophyceae*. It may be more commonly known as Irish moss. It is used in the cosmetic industry to stabilise emulsions, and is a thickener and viscocity increasing agent. This edible red seaweed, which is used in the food industry as well, has been used in medicines in India for many years, but only became a popular food ingredient at the onset of World War II during which it was used instead of agar-agar.

CITRIC ACID is a water-soluble organic acid found in many fruits especially citrus fruits. It is used in cosmetic products as a pH adjuster and chelating substance. (See also **ALPHA-HYDROXY ACIDS**.)

CITRUS DULCIS is the EU-labelling name for a variety of extracts and derivatives obtained from the orange *Citrus aurantium var. dulcis*. Orange extract is obtained from the fruit of this orange, which was native to the Indo-Malayan region and China, but is now widely cultivated in many tropical and subtropical areas of the world. It has a high percentage of Vitamin C. Orange seed extract is derived from the seeds of this orange; a peel extract and a peel wax is obtained from the peel; orange flower extract comes from the flowers; and orange flower oil is the volatile oil expressed from the flowers. Another volatile orange oil is extracted from a different species, *Citrus sinesis*. This is the sweet orange, the best known of all citrus fruits. To extract the oil, the fresh peel from the sweet orange fruit is crushed. Materials extracted from the orange are used in cosmetics to make

the product smell good, and are harmless (except that berga-
mot oil, from *Citrus bergamia*, another species, is sensitive to
oxidation and should not be used in sunscreen products).

CITRUS GRANDIS is the EU-labelling name for a variety of extracts and derivatives obtained from the grapefruit
Citrus grandis. Grapefruit extract is produced from the fruit
of the citrus plant – it contains Vitamin C and has antiseptic
properties that are said to help in relieving an oily skin.
Grapefruit seed extract is extracted from the seeds of *Citrus
grandis*. The seeds have antibacterial properties. Grapefruit
leaf extract is obtained from the crushed leaves; grapefruit
juice is the actual fluid that results when the pulp of fresh
grapefruit is crushed. Extract from the juice is more beneficial
than that of the rind, which contains little Vitamin C and is
subjected to environmental influences such as pesticides and
fertilisers, which in turn can lead to sensitivity. Grapefruit
peel extract comes from the peel.

CI 42053 relates to a colour additive. (See below item and
COLOURS.)

CI 75120. (See **ANNATTO**.) CI, meaning Colour Index,
followed by a number indicates a particular colour has been
added to a product. The colour annatto is CI 75120.

CI 77007. (See above item and **ULTRAMARINES**.)

COCAMIDE DEA. This is the old name for **COCONUT
DEA** (see below).

COCAMIDOPROPYL BETAINE is basically a synthetic
substance that derives from coconut oil, and is used in liquid
soaps as an anti-static agent, surfactant, skin conditioning
agent, viscosity increasing agent, cleansing ingredient and
foam booster.

COCOATE. (See **SODIUM COCOATE**.)

COCO-CAPRYLATE/CAPRATE is a combination of
coconut alcohol esters of capric acid and caprylic acid. It is
used in cosmetics for skin conditioning and emollient
purposes.

COCOGLUCOSIDE is a surfactant often used in effervescent bath tablets and balls.

COCONUT DEA (DEA is diethanolamide) is the

diethanolamide of coconut acid. Produced by reacting diethanolamine with coconut fatty acid, it forms neutral soaps and is used as thickeners and detergents.

COCOS NUCIFERA (coconut oil). This highly saturated fat is obtained by crushing the kernels of the seeds of the coconut palm, *Cocos nucifera*. It is used extensively in the manufacture of soap and skin cleansers. This oil is another particularly rich emollient that does not go as rancid as some others when exposed to the air. It is excellent for massage creams for this reason. Technical names include coconut oil and copra oil.

COLA ACUMINATA (cola or kola nut extract). The seeds of the *Cola acuminata* tree, which originated in tropical Africa but which is now widely cultivated in South America, contain stimulants caffeine, tannin and theobromine, which are useful in counteracting fatigue. With regard to cosmetics, they have astringent, stimulating, healing, anti-inflammatory and anti-irritant properties.

COLLAGEN is a fibrous protein derived from animal cartilage and other connective tissue. It has high moisture retention properties so is therefore ideal for many skin care formulations, particularly moisturisers. It is one of the cheapest, most effective proteins used in the industry. Collagen helps to reduce natural moisture loss by forming a film on the skin. It is said to improve elasticity and help combat dry skin, making it smooth and soft. It is similar to the collagen produced in the skin and bones of the body, and is often obtained from the skin of calves.

COLLOIDAL MAGNESIUM ALUMINIUM SILICATE is obtained from natural smectite clays and used as thickeners in products such as creams and lotions as well as toothpastes, cosmetics, and shampoos. It has an excellent stabilising ability.

COLOURS. Extensively used in cosmetics, colours may be animal, vegetable or mineral derived. They are not essential but are generally added to attract the consumer. For example, when purchasing a cucumber hand cream, the addition of a gentle pastel green would suggest the properties of that fine green fellow were in the pot in its succulent, cooling form. Add to that a touch of a cucumber synthetic aromatic ingredient and stand by the till. Cosmetic manufacturers have to find a safe, stable as well as attractive colour. Most often synthetics are used. There are two types – dyes and pigments. Dyes are soluble in water or oil. They are used to colour the product itself, for example, in a shampoo, cream or bath foam. Pigments are insoluble in either water or oil. They are used to colour the skin or eyelashes and are found in colour cosmetics such as eyeshadow, lipstick and rouge. Pigments may be a single chemical (for example, iron oxides which can be black, brown, red or yellow) or could be a dye as above, rendered insoluble by depositing it on an insoluble substrate such as talc or aluminium oxide.

It is important to be aware that even if a dye or pigment is allowed for cosmetic use there may be restrictions on the type of product it can be used in. Different countries have different regulations regarding the use of colours in cosmetics. Generally a Colour Index (CI) number on the label indicates the colour used in a cosmetic product. There are 116 permitted certified colours available for cosmetic formulators to use. On labels, if you see the sign +/- followed by a colour, it means 'may contain'. Animal-derived colours include crimson cochineal (see **CARMINE**), gained by crushing the bodies of cactus-chewing cochineal insects which are found in Mexico, the Canary Islands and other places where cacti grow. Pearl essences are formed from fish scale or bismuth oxychloride, and manganese violet. Vegetable colourings commonly used in cosmetics are beet, grape skin, beta carotene and caramel. Plant-derived colours include annatto (a yellowish-red dye which comes from the seeds of a small tropical American tree); carotene (present in many plants); the green chlorophyll (E140, obtained from plants); turmeric (from a tropical Asian plant called *Curcuma longa*); and saffron (an Eastern hemisphere crocus with orange stigmas which are used as a colorant). Inorganic colours include titanium dioxide, barium sulphate, zinc oxide, iron oxide, bronze powder, ultramarines and chromium oxide greens. Colours rarely cause skin reactions such as dermatitis, but there have been reports of this occurring when coal dyes are used.

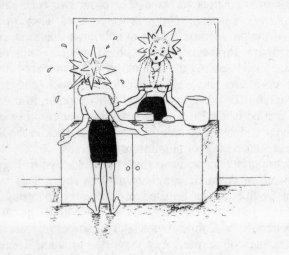

Twenty minutes later my hair was quite white!

Maurene writes: Digressing slightly now, but I thought I'd share the following experience with you. On one of those days when I was bored with the world in general and myself in particular, I decided to change my image and try a new hair colour. The fact that gentlemen prefer blondes made me decide to become one. I bought a packet of powdered bleach, made it up as directed and applied it. Twenty minutes later my hair was quite white! As I was due to fly out to Africa that evening on duty, something had to be done fast. I frantically applied a light brown toner – which simply turned the hair a tomato colour with a halo of green. Panic set in, for the airline I worked for supplied the cabin staff with delightful mauve uniforms. Envisaging the colour scheme of tomato red, brilliant green and mauve propelled me down the road to where I knew a hairdresser lived, although I had never met her. With my tresses wrapped in a towel I knocked on her door and found her to be extremely sympathetic but she could only direct me to the nearest salon which would have the suitable products needed to correct my disaster. A few days later I called in with a bottle of wine to thank her. She told me that when I first called she had been suffering from a bout of depression but the sight of my hair coupled with the fact I was only a few hours away from attending a jet load of passengers had been the turning point in her recovery. (Gentlemen can prefer blondes if they like, but I am going to stay mousey).

COPERNICIA CERIFERA (carnauba wax). The wax is derived from the Brazilian Carnauba palm tree, *Copernicia cerifera*. Its large palmate leaves and leaf buds are laden with a covering of wax. When the tree is shaken, the wax falls to the ground where it is gathered and later processed. There are three colours (brown, yellow and 'fatty' grey), which vary according to the age of the leaves. Carnauba wax is commonly used for coating tablets, furniture polish, scented candles, and in cosmetics it is used in mascara, hair-care preparations, creams and deodorants.

CORN OIL. (See **ZEA MAYS**.)

CORN STARCH is obtained from corn or maize kernels, *Zea mays*. In cosmetics and face powders it is used as a thickener. Corn starch absorbs water and is soothing to the skin.

CORYLUS AVELLANA (hazelnut oil) is produced almost everywhere in Europe but the carefully selected fruits grown to well defined specifications are mainly cultivated in the Mediterranean region. The oil is expressed from the nuts of the hazelnut tree, *Corylus avellana*. Hazelnut and sweet almond oil have the same components, their stability is identical and they have the same properties. However, the diffusion and penetration powers of hazelnut oil are higher than those of the latter. In addition, no greasy feeling occurs when it is applied to the skin. Due to its percentage of monounsaturated fatty acids (82 per cent oleic acid), it has a better stability against autoxidation and therefore a better shelf life than those with a higher degree of polyunsaturated fatty acids.

COTTON SEED OIL. (See **GOSSYPIUM**.)

CRYSTALLINE CAMPHOR. Crude camphor is extracted in crystalline form from *Cinnamomum camphora* trees. After processing, it is used predominantly in pre-shave and aftershave lotions and skin fresheners. It is credited with having cooling, antiseptic and refreshing properties.

CUCUMIS SATIVUS (cucumber juice) is the juice extracted from the vegetable *Cucumis sativus* for its soothing, refreshing, moisture regulating and anti-inflammatory properties. It contains amino and organic acids, minerals and mucins (glycoproteins – substances in plants that cement cells together). It is beneficial in aftershave and eye products, and is used in products for balancing oily skin. Cucumber oil is the fixed oil obtained from the same species of cucumber (*Cucumis sativus)* by expression.

CURCUMA LONGA (turmeric) is an extract or a powder derived from *Curcuma longa,* commonly known as turmeric. Natives of India have used the rhizomes of turmeric for centuries as a medicine, spice and colouring agent. It is now cultivated widely throughout the world. It is used in cosmetics for its skin soothing properties.

CYCLOMETHICONES are a family of cyclic silicone derivatives, a group of non-tacky materials that can deliver active ingredients and also serve as a vehicle for carrying fragrance. They are used in skin products for the silky smooth feel their conditioning agent gives.

DAUCUS CAROTA is the EU-labelling name given to various extracts and derivatives of the ordinary garden carrot, *Daucus carota.* It is rich in carotene, a compound that is converted into Vitamin A by the liver. It has been used since the Dark Ages for skin diseases and is still used today for relieving acne, dermatitis, and rashes. Carrot juice is the actual liquid that results when the fresh flesh of the carrot *Daucus carota sativa* is pressed. Carrot oil is expressed from the crushed seeds of this carrot.

DEA is an abbreviation of diethanolamide. See **DIETH-ANOLAMIDE**.

DEA-CETYL PHOSPHATE is an organic salt derived from phosphorous compounds, used as a surfactant and emulsifying agent.

DECETH 8 belongs to the chemical class alkoxylated alcohols. It is a surfactant and emulsifying agent.

DECYL ALCOHOL is derived commercially from liquid paraffin and occurs naturally in sweet orange and ambrette seed. It is an antifoam agent, a fixative in perfumes and acts as an intermediate for surface-active agents.

DECYL OLEATE is an ester, an emollient that is absorbed by the skin easily, allowing the product to be spread efficiently so giving a pleasant feel to the skin. It is a component of the sebum of human skin, and is also produced synthetically from olive oil.

DEIONISED WATER – water from which the ions (electrically charged atoms) of water hardness have been removed.

DILAURYL THIODIPROPIONATE – an antioxidant.

DICAPRYLATE DICAPRATE (glycerides) is used in bath oils to help leave the skin feeling soft and smooth.

DICAPRYLYL ETHER is an ether used for its skin conditioning action.

DICHLOROBENZYL ALCOHOL is a preservative and biocide.

DIETHANOLAMIDE is a chemical used in shaving creams to make the product foam and thicken.

DIHYDROXYACETONE. This is a chemical skin tan agent used in artificial tanning preparations to make the skin simulate a suntan.

DIMETHICONE is a form of silicone that is incorporated into skin care products to impart lubrication, slip and a non-tacky feel. It is used as a base ingredient in ointments, as a topical drug vehicle and to protect the skin against moisture loss when used in larger quantities. In combination with other ingredients it is a useful waterproofing material for sunscreen emulsions. It also helps to decrease the greasiness that high sun protection factor (SPF) products often contain. Dimethicone helps to improve the durability of some substances on the skin.

DIMETHICONE COPOLYOL is a polymer of a mixture of silicone compounds. It is used as a skin conditioning agent.

DIMETHICONOL is a silicone derivative with affinity for water. It is used as an anti-foaming agent, skin conditioning agent and emollient.

DIMETHICONOL ESTERS – fatty wax that liquifies when rubbed on the skin.

DIOCTYL MALEATE – an ester derived from malic acid. It is a skin conditioning agent and emollient.

DIOCTYL SODIUM SULPHOSUCCINATE. This sodium salt is used in cosmetics as a surfactant and cleansing agent.

DIOSCOREA VILLOSA (wild yam). Extracts from the wild yam *Dioscorea villosa* are used in cosmetics today, although for the last two hundred years wild yam has been used by many cultures for complaints such as gallbladder pain, painful menstruation and to lower blood pressure. Mexican women have been using wild yam as a contraceptive for centuries, and one of today's birth control pills is made from the wild yam. The plant is grown extensively in mid-western and eastern USA, Mexico and Asia. It is used in cosmetics for its claimed anti-inflammatory and antioxidant properties.

DIPROPYLENE GLYCOL is the di-ether of propylene glycol and is used as a solvent, as a viscosity-decreasing agent and for moisturising purposes.

DISODIUM EDTA is a substituted amino acid; a chelating agent (see Glossary) in cosmetics.

DISTEARATE SODIUM is a surfactant.

DJARAK IRI OIL. Originating from Indonesia, this is practically colourless and odourless and contains mainly ricinoleic acid and linoleic acid. The oil is a natural blend of castor and curcas oil and is obtained by pressing together the seeds of the castor and curcas plants, which look very much alike. However, the oils of both plants have very different compositions.

DROMICEIUS is emu oil, which may be known by one of its trade names, kalaya oil. It is a recent introduction to the modern cosmetics world, although the Australian Aborigines have used it for thousands of years as a protective and softening emollient on the skin, for joint and muscle pain and to ease inflammation. Emu oil is extracted from the fat of the emu bird, *Domaius novaehollandiae*. Apparently, on specialised emu rearing farms their diets are strictly controlled without the use of pesticides, insecticides or anthelmintics (drugs used to destroy intestinal worms). The high oleic acid content of emu oil makes it ideal for use in skin creams, bath products, shower gels, shampoos and medicated soap – it's good for sensitive skins as it does not dry out the skin.

ELAEIS GUINEENSIS (palm kernel oil). The *Elaeis guineensis* palm, native to West Africa, is now grown in plantations in south-east Asia, Malaysia, equatorial and West Africa and in certain parts of Brazil. The oil is extracted from the seeds of the palm tree and is used to make soap products including baby soaps, as well as ointments. Palm oil is also used by natives of all countries for cooking and personal grooming. The palm seeds, with a fat content of 40-50 per cent, are removed from the soft reddish-yellow fruit and the oil is obtained by pressing and extraction. A palm kernel wax is produced from palm kernel oil.

ELASTIN is an animal-derived protein, said to help retain moisture, relieve dryness and give the skin a feeling of flexibility and smoothness. For cosmetic products use, it is generally obtained from bovine neck ligaments. It is mainly used as a surface protective agent and in products for mature skin. Elastin and collagen are both proteins found in the dermis. They are similar in composition, although elastin has different amino acids and is found in lower concentrations. Also, elastin molecules are smaller hence the ability to penetrate the surface epidermal layers and subsequently improve skin appearance.

EMBRYO EXTRACT is extracted from mammalian embryo skin, such as foetal calves, for a special hormone that is said to restore skin to a more youthful looking age.

However, this is a grey area in which some scientists agree with the theory, while others do not. It is used mainly in so-called 'anti-ageing' creams.

EMU OIL. (See **DROMICEIUS**.)

EMULSIFIERS. These are agents that help to create an emulsion. They hold water-based and oil-based ingredients together. They assist in keeping the product properly mixed, uniform and smooth. (An emulsion in this context is a mixture in which an oily substance is dispersed in another liquid, usually in water but can also be a dispersion of water-in-oil.)

EMULSIFYING WAX. This is not really a wax – rather it is a combination of fatty alcohol and emulsifiers which, when mixed with water, blend together to make a cream.

ENZYMES are catalysts that come from vegetable or animal origin. They enable a biochemical change to take place. In cosmetics, common enzymes include amylase and chymotrypsin, and superoxide dismutase, the latter of which is known as a free radical reducing enzyme.

ESSENTIAL FATTY ACIDS form the basic building blocks of body fats and cellular membranes. They are one of a group of unsaturated fatty acids that are essential for growth but cannot be synthesized by the body.

ESSENTIAL OILS are volatile, aromatic substances found in a wide range of plants. They derive from flowers, leaves, fruits, seeds, rhizomes, roots, resins, petals and barks. They are extracted by steam, water, short-path (or molecular) or dry distillation, enfleurage (an ancient method which is generally obsolete but still used for very expensive fragrances), solvent expression (where chemicals are used to extract the oil), maceration (where flowers are soaked in hot fixed oil and filtered) and mechanical expression. The latter method is mainly applicable to citrus fruit peels. Yonks ago, lemon oil was expressed by hand, using sponges to soak up the oil which was then squeezed out. Today the oil is obtained by abrading the peel in machines or it comes as a by-product of the fruit juice trade.

Essential oils should be of high quality. Those containing

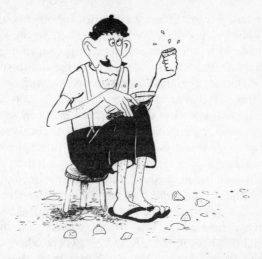

Yonks ago, lemon oil was expressed by hand, using sponges to soak up the oil which was then squeezed out.

synthesized fragrance chemicals may increase the chances of skin sensitivity and allergic reactions ranging from subtle discomfort to persistent inflammation. Even high quality essential oils should not be used neat, particularly in the bath. A few drops of the wrong oil in a bath may cause skin irritation because of the little understood fact that essential oils and water *do not mix*. When a few drops of oil are put into the bathwater and agitated, they appear to mix but in fact both the oil molecules and the water molecules will soon be attracted back to their own family. So, should you sit upon a blob of undiluted oil in the tub it may just find an orifice into which it may take an unwelcome peek! Ginger, lemon and other citrus oils, lemongrass, thyme, peppermint and a few others can cause irritation and, in excess, damage to delicate mucous membranes and the eyes. Follow instructions carefully, buy a bath product where the oil is already dispersed, or dilute the essential oil with full cream milk.

Few essential oils sold are from one single botanical source. To be commercially viable the same named oil may be purchased from different countries (or other sources in the same country) and then blended together, so the Latin name applicable to a particular sub-species grown in one area will not apply to the mixed oil. Each of these sub-species will have different chemical constituents varying in chemical properties. However, fear ye botanically not. There are advantages in knowing the difference between some botanicals, a good example being from the eucalyptus genus. *Eucalyptus globulus* is known to help in respiratory upsets whereas *Eucalyptus citriodora* – with its lemon odour – is mentally unwinding without the sedative effect of lavender. One lavender, *Lavandula angustifolia*, has twelve cultivars, each with a different name and varying chemical constituents! However, there are a few small growers and distillers of essential oils both in the UK and elsewhere where oils can be obtained from source. Oils purchased from them are more likely to be of just one botanic species, but beware those that claim, 'Every flower is picked by hand with loving care'; this is a good sign of either a con merchant or a supplier who knows nothing about essential oil production. Only a few oils are produced from hand picked flowers, the harvesters are often on piece work and pick at first light, so forget about the loving care, it's more likely to be, 'The quicker I get these flowers in, the sooner I can go back to bed'. Most essential oil bearing plants are produced as agricultural crops due to the huge volumes of plant material necessary for the extraction of essential oils. Many plants yield less than 1 per cent of essential oil and even lavender may only yield 2-8 per cent of the total plant mass depending on the variety.

Some essential oils are not generally acceptable to the olfactory nerves (the ones you sniff with) such as garlic. Garlic contains about 0.2 per cent of a pungent-smelling essential oil with superb anti-bacterial properties. The ancient Egyptians considered garlic a vital part of the wages given to labourers building the pyramids and one of the first recorded strikes was by workers on the Kings' tombs who were not being supplied with enough food including their garlic. Roman foot soldiers were issued with a clove of garlic a day to maintain good health. Remember though, that one man's meat is another's poison – an essential oil which suits one person may be an allergen to another.

ESTERS. This embraces a wide range of organic compounds varying in properties and usage. They are formed from the reaction between an alcohol and an organic acid. There are hundreds upon hundreds of such materials, from isopropyl myristate, used in emollient giving situations in skin care, through to ethyl acetate.

ETHYLENE BRASSYLATE is an ester.

ETHYLPARABEN is an ester and phenol, used as a preservative.

EXTRA CELLULAR MATRIX is a combination of collagen, sulphates, glycoproteins, glycosaminoglycans, and other bioactive substances that are said to stimulate and repair skin cells. It is used particularly in products for mature skin.

FARNESOL is an organic compound (sesquiterpene alcohol) found in vegetables and many essential oils such as rose, cumin, cinnamon and hops. It is used in perfumery to enhance sweet floral odours as well as in cosmetics where it is said to help retain moisture within the skin. It is now also extensively used in Europe as a nature identical bacteriostatic agent in aerosols, sticks and roll-on deodorants.

FATS. (See **OILS, FATS AND WAXES**.)

FATTY ACID ESTERS are emollients and emulsifiers used in hand and general skin care products because of their oily yet non-greasy consistency when rubbed into the skin.

FIBRONECTIN. Made from animal blood, this fibrous glycoprotein strengthens the skin's connective tissues and membranes. It is found in connective tissues, membranes and in plasma. It is believed to encourage cell growth, and may even regenerate cells. In cosmetics it is used for moisturising and defending the skin, and maintaining the basal layer in particular.

FLOWER WAXES. These waxy substances, obtained from sources such as mimosa, lavender, orange, jasmine and rose flowers, remain once the essential oil has been distilled from the fresh plant material. Sometimes the waste product is treated with alcohol and then with water to ensure every usable portion is extracted. This residue is sometimes sold and for a high price, considering there is not much of the original product left. The waxes do manage to give creams and lotions a subtle scent and have superb emollience.

FORMALDEHYDE. (See **PRESERVATIVES**.)

FRAGRANCE. Smell is an important aspect of any cosmetic, so this is carefully chosen by manufacturers and marketing experts to suit the product, current trends and the target market. Natural and synthetic fragrances are used.

GAMMA-ORYZANOL is the ester of ferulic acid (an organic compound) and terpene alcohol. It is used in perfumes.

GELATIN is extracted from collagen, which comes from the bones, skin and white connective tissues of mammals. It is obtained by partial hydrolysis.

GINSENG. (See **PANAX GINSENG EXTRACT**.)

GLA (**GAMMA LINOLENIC ACID**) is important for a healthy body. It can be made in the human body from the essential fatty acid known as linoleic acid, which is found in certain food. Studies have shown that the conversion of linoleic acid into gamma linolenic acid in the body tissues can be inhibited and this can lead to abnormally low levels of certain prostaglandins (see Glossary) which regulate many bodily functions. It can be inhibited by processed oils, fats, margarines and cholesterols, low zinc, low insulin, excess alcohol, certain viruses and ageing. Therapeutically GLA is used for many conditions. It is said to help to: improve blood circulation; relieve pre-menstrual pains; counteract specific disorders such as hyperactivity (in children), male impotence and multiple sclerosis; slow down the effects of ageing; revitalise dry skin; and counteract the harmful effects of too many high-meat-processed-food diets. GLA is therefore added to many dietary supplements, cosmetic products, infant nutrition products, animal nutrition products, and pure GLA is used as a precursor to prostaglandins.

GLYCERINE (a technical name for this is **glycerol**) is a colourless, odourless, syrupy liquid, sweet in taste. It occurs in combination with fatty acids in animal and vegetable fats and oils. It is a by-product of soap manufacture and it is used as a solvent, plasticizer and sweetener. Some glycerine is also obtained by fermentation of sugars.

GLYCEROL. (See **GLYCERINE**.)

GLYCEROL STEARATE is solid ester formed from glycerine and stearic acid and is used as a thickener/ stabiliser in creams. A modified (self-emulsifying) version is very commonly used as the emulsifier in creams and lotions.

GLYCERYL COCOATE – an emulsifier and skin conditioning material derived from coconut oil. 'Glyceryl' is a way of describing the compound formed from the alcohol glycerol and some acid.

GLYCERYL OLEATE is the ester from glycerine and oleic acid and is a skin conditioning agent.

GLYCERYL STEARATE – an emulsifier made from glycerine and stearic fatty acids, which helps in forming neutral and stable emulsions. For cosmetic use it is derived from palm kernel or soya oil and is used as a skin conditioning material.

GLYCINE SOJA (soybean oil). The oil is extracted from the seeds of the soybean legume called *Glycine soja* that is cultivated worldwide but particularly in the USA, China, Japan and Asia. It is a skin conditioning material used in cosmetic products such as bath oils, soaps and shampoos.

GLYCINE. This is a white, sweet, crystalline amino acid that is found in most proteins. In cosmetics it is used as an anti-static agent, buffering agent and skin conditioning agent.

GLYCOL STEARATE is one of the most widely used bases for cosmetic creams. It is the ester of ethylene glycol and stearic acid. It changes clear cleansers to pearly ones and can be used as a detergent, emulsifier, surfactant, thickener, stabiliser and emollient in cosmetic formulations.

GLYCOLCOPOLYMERS. These are silicone derivatives with an affinity for water. They can leave a deposit on the surface of bath water and subsequently make the skin feel soft and smooth.

GLYCOLIC ACID is an organic alpha-hydroxy acid and is found in sugar cane. It is popular with cosmetic formulators as it penetrates layers of dead skin, which it dissolves. In doing so it can clear an acne-covered skin, reduce fine wrinkles of sun-damaged skin, and lessen the dark pigmentation of liver spots (actinic keratosis).

GLYCOLS are a group of polyhydric (meaning many oxygen and hydrogen groups) alcohols used extensively in cosmetics as humectants. Glycerine is a polyhydric alcohol. Propylene glycol and glycerine are popularly used glycols.

GLYCOSAMINOGLYCAN (also known as mucopolysaccharide) – any one of a group of polysaccharides that contain amino sugars. These are extracted from varying animal tissues including shark and bovine cartilage and placenta, and have elastic properties. These skin conditioning materials have superior moisturising and regenerative properties.

GLYCYRRHIZA GLABRA (liquorice) is extracted from the roots and stem of the liquorice plant *Glycyrrhiza glabra* for its skin soothing and softening properties. It possibly absorbs UV rays as well as having a de-pigmenting effect and an inhibitory effect on the synthesis of melanin.

GOLD OF PLEASURE OIL. (See **CAMELINA SATIVA**.)

GOSSYPIUM (cotton seed oil) is a by-product of the cotton industry. The oil is extracted from the seeds of different species of cotton (*Gossypium* family) after the fibres and seeds have been separated in a cotton gin. It is widely used in cosmetics as a fixed oil and in soaps, baby products and cream.

HAMAMELIS VIRGINIANA (witch hazel) is extracted from the bark and leaves of the North American plant *Hamamelis virginiana*. A biological additive, it is widely used as an astringent and skin freshener. Witch hazel contains between 70 to 80 per cent ethanol and between 2 to 9 per cent tannin, although the witch hazel water one usually buys over the counter has an ethanol content of 15 per cent.

HAZELNUT OIL. (See **CORYLUS AVELLANA.**)

HELIANTHUS ANNUUS is the EU-labelling name given to extracts of the sunflower, *Helianthus annuus*. Sunflower extract is taken from the whole sunflower; sunflower seed extract is obtained from its seeds; sunflower oil is expressed from its seeds (and, incidentally, is second only to soybean as a worldwide source of edible vegetable oil). The fraction of the seed oil that is not saponified during the refining process is known as seed oil unsaponifiables. See Glossary. Helianthus Annuus is used in the cosmetic industry for it is a very rich emollient with a high content of Vitamin E.

HIPPOPHAE RHAMNOIDES (sea buckthorn). This extract comes from the fruit of the sea buckthorn *Hippophae rhamnoides*, a Eurasian maritime shrub that yields orange-red edible berries. The extract is a natural bactericide, antioxidant and analgesic. An oil is extracted from the kernels of the plant. Tibetans use the oil to relieve rheumatism. It may also be used in topical applications to improve cell metabolism of subcutaneous tissue and as a free radical scavenger to help delay dermal ageing processes.

HONEY. (See **MEL.**)

HOPLOSTETHUS (Orange Roughy Oil). This is not the oil extracted from a rough orange as one may expect, but is the oil obtained from the fat under the skin of a deep-sea fish known as *Hoplostethus atlanticus*. It is used in skin care preparations because of its good spreading and skin softening capabilities. Orange Roughy Oil is its technical name.

HORDEUM VULGARE (barley). The oil is extracted from the seeds of the barley plant *Hordeum vulgare* and is used mainly as a fixed oil, which contains soothing properties. The oil is used by herbalists to treat intestinal problems. Waxes are made out of the spent barley grain for use as emollients.

HUMAN PLACENTAL ENZYMES, HUMAN PLACENTAL LIPIDS, AND **HUMAN PLACENTAL PROTEIN** are extracted from healthy human placentas for use in cosmetics as skin conditioning materials. These ingredients are now banned in the EU, but some other countries still use them.

HUMECTANTS are substances that are by nature hygroscopic, that is, they will absorb moisture from the air or solutions. The best example is glycerine (glycerol) which absorbs up to 50 per cent of its weight of water vapour. Another popular humectant is sorbitol, which used to be prepared from the sugar from rowan berries and other fruits of the *Rosaceae* family, but now only a synthetic sorbitol is produced industrially.

HYALURONIC ACID can be an animal-derived protein used as a moisturising substance. Originally it was extracted only from cocks' combs and other animal sources, but now there is also a similar plant-derived alternative. It is also present in the liquid surrounding joints of the body. Hyaluronic acid is a natural mucopolysaccharide (glycosaminoglycan).

HYDROCARBONS. Organic compounds consisting of only carbon and hydrogen. Hydrocarbon products, including paraffin wax, petrolatum and mineral oils, are used in the production of hand and body lotions and sunscreens but are losing favour, increasingly being replaced by emollient esters of fatty acids.

HYDROGEN PEROXIDE is a colourless, unstable liquid which releases oxygen when it breaks down. It is used in cosmetics as a skin bleach, and is perhaps more commonly known for being applied to the hair for bleaching it white (blonde).

HYDROGENATED COCO GLYCERIDES. Deriving from coconut oil, this is a skin conditioning ingredient.

HYDROGENATED PALM GLYCERIDES. Deriving from palm oil, this is an ester type of substance used as a skin conditioning agent.

HYDROGENATED POLYISOBUTENE is an emollient.

HYDROGENATED VEGETABLE GLYCERIDES CITRATE is a citric acid ester and is a skin conditioning ingredient.

HYDROGENATED VEGETABLE OIL. Vegetable oils are obtained from plants such as peanut, sesame, olive and cottonseed. They are used in many cosmetic preparations.

Hydrogenated fats are often used as inexpensive bulking components in various formulations. Their properties are easily changed by adjusting the degree of hydrogenation (see Glossary).

HYDROQUINONE is a natural white, crystalline, solid phenol although much is now made synthetically. It is an antioxidant pigment lightening cream used in skin bleaching creams, freckle creams and suntan lotions. When it is exposed to air it turns brown. Long-term use of bleach creams can result in ochronosis – where the skin and other body tissues become discoloured brown. Used in high concentration it causes unpleasant reactions. It is now prohibited in skin lightening preparations.

HYDROXYETHYLCELLULOSE is a gum used as an emulsion stabiliser and binder.

HYDROXYPROPYL METHYLCELLULOSE is a gum used as an emulsion stabiliser.

HYPERICUM PERFORATUM EXTRACT (St John's wort). This oil is extracted from the flowering tops of this shrubby, perennial plant (*Hypericum perforatum)* that likes dry, gravelly soils. It grows in sunny places in many parts of the world, including eastern North America and the Pacific coast. The oil extract is used for relieving burns, sores, insect bites and other skin problems and is incorporated into many cosmetics, including sun products, hand and face creams and baby skin care products.

IMIDAZOLIDINYL UREA. (See **PRESERVATIVES**.)

IODOPROPYNYL BUTYLCARBAMATE is an organic compound, used as a preservative.

IRON OXIDE is an inorganic compound, used in cosmetics as a colour additive.

ISOBUTYLPARABEN is an ester and phenol, used in cosmetics as a preservative. Part of the paraben group of preservatives. (See also **PRESERVATIVES**.)

ISOCETYL STEARATE is an ester and is used as a skin conditioner.

ISOHEXADECANE is a hydrocarbon, and functions in cosmetics as a skin conditioning agent.

ISOPROPYL ALCOHOL. This antibacterial alcohol changes the nature of certain components. It is made from propylene, which results when petroleum is broken down in a particular way. It has been used in lotions, aftershave lotions and as a solvent for essential oils but it is no longer commonly used because of its odour which is difficult to mask. It is also a denaturant, anti-foaming agent and viscosity decreasing agent.

ISOPROPYL ISOSTEARATE is an ester of an alcohol and an acid. An emollient and a skin conditioner.

ISOPROPYL MYRISTATE is derived from isopropyl alcohol and myristic acid. This widely used ingredient has been found to cause comedones (blackheads) in some formulations. Some cosmetic manufacturers use an alternative or, having tested their product effectively, generally add 'non-comedogenic' to the product's label. It is low viscosity oil, leaves a good feel to the skin, and is often found in insect repellents.

ISOPROPYL PALMITATE is often derived from coconut for use as an emollient and moisturiser. It is an ester produced by combining palmitic acid and isopropyl alcohol.

ISOPROPYLBENZYL SALICYLATE is a UV absorber which is added to sun care products to help prevent sunburn.

ISOSTEARIC ACID is a fatty acid, used in skin care preparations as a cleansing agent and surfactant.

ISOSTEARYL NEOPENTANOATE is an ester, used for skin conditioning and as an emollient.

JAPAN WAX. (See **RHUS SUCCEDANEA**.)

JOJOBA EXTRACT. (See **BUXUS CHINENSIS**.)

JUNIPERUS COMMUNIS is the EU-labelling name given to an extract and an essential oil derived from the juniper bush (or small tree) *Juniperus communis* of the *Cupressaceae* family. Juniperus communis extract comes from the ripe fruit of this tree, and Juniperus communis oil is the essential oil extracted from the berries. It is used in soaps and perfumes as a fragrance additive, and it is claimed by some manufacturers to be good for oily and acned skins as it contains anti-bacterial properties.

KAOLIN (also known as china clay) is a fine, white clay consisting of a variety of aluminium magnesium silicates. It is used in the porcelain and bone china industry as well as in emollients and face masques to help absorb oily or sweaty deposits on the skin.

KERATIN is the fibrous protein found in our hair, skin and nails. For cosmetic purposes it is usually obtained from hydrolyzed bovine horn, horsehair and the bristles on boars' backs. It comes in a brown powder form so is easy for formulators to add it to products. It is used as a skin conditioning agent. (See also **BIOLOGICAL ADDITIVES**.)

KEROSENE (deodorised) may be found in heavy-duty hand cleansers. It is derived from petroleum but has been de-coloured and deodorised by being washed with fuming sulphuric acid (a mixture of acids). Generally, it irritates the skin which can result in dermatitis, but when used in cosmetics it is considerably diluted and therefore harmless. Because of its solvent action on fats it can cause dry skin.

KIWI SEED OIL. (See **ACTINIDIA CHINENSIS**.)

KOJIC ACID MONOSTEARATE is derived from kojic acid, a skin lightening agent common in Japan. Research has discovered that it tends to decrease the production of the enzyme tyrosinase in the skin and therefore melanin formation, making it suitable for use in skin bleaching cosmetics.

LACTIC ACID is an organic acid used in skin fresheners (toners) for its acidic properties. It is normally found in the body and consists of metabolised glucose and glycogen, formed by the fermentation of sugars by the lactobacilli and some moulds. It is an AHA (alpha-hydroxy acid) occurring in sour milk and other foods. It has the ability to hold moisture and improve pliability within the stratum corneum. It is also a pH adjuster.

LANOLIN ALCOHOLS can also be known as sterols, triterpene alcohols and aliphatic alcohols. They derive from lanolin and are extensively used as emulsifiers and emollients in hand creams and lotions.

LANOLIN CERA (lanolin wax). (From *lana* meaning wool and *oleum* meaning oil in Latin). This yellowish viscous wax is obtained by refining the wool grease that is secreted by the sebaceous glands of sheep. Wool grease provides the fleece with a protective coating. The excess oils and sebum excreted by the animals' oil glands are removed and the waxes are fractionated out by molecular distillation. A rumpus was caused in the 1970s when it was decided that lanolin was a common allergen found in cosmetics, despite it having been used as an emollient for skin problems for three thousand years. However, research in the 1980s proved that this was probably less of an allergen than many accepted foods. Lanolin moisturises partly by slight occlusion but mainly by penetrating the stratum corneum, down to the stratum granulosum. Here it holds the moisture (like a reservoir) which can be released to the skin's dry outer layer when necessary and so hydrates the skin, keeping it smooth and reducing the possibility of invasion by bacteria or viruses by closing cracks which occur with dry skin. It basically protects human skin in much the same way as the wax on the sheep's wool protects the animal from the ravages of severe weather and climatic conditions.

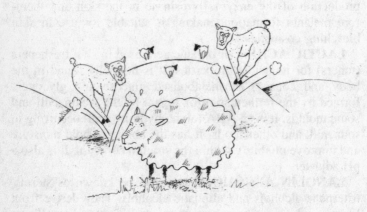

The sheep are absolutely delighted to get rid of their woolly overcoats.

There is no cruelty involved in shearing their woolly coats off – in fact, come summer the sheepies are absolutely delighted to get rid of their woolly overcoats. Not only do Mr and Mrs Baa get relief from overheating, they also have less weight to carry around. Sheep which remain unshorn are at much more risk from the breeding habits of the blow fly, as the wool is an excellent medium in which flies lay their eggs, the end result of which is an invasion of maggots which dine off the animals' flesh.

Interestingly, the hands and arms of shepherds and others working with sheep are renowned for being delightfully soft. The possessors of such velvety skin have to be very careful while in a darkened theatre or cinema when a sudden moment of drama could result in the inadvertent clutching of a hand; the clutcher being deluded into thinking such a hand must be that of the opposite sex. Perchance shepherds should watch more than their flocks by night!

In Roman times 'her indoors' used to plaster herself with raw, untreated lanolin, most reminiscent of Dominus and Domina Sheep, and so bedecked went to the bed chamber. 'Him indoors' had to endure the night sleeping (or trying to) beside this odiferous better half. She, on awakening and completing her toilette, would have silken, sensuous to the touch skin, ready to spend amorous hours with her latest lover. Vive les Roman fair persons! Incidentally, lanolin sold in ancient Rome was called Athenian Oesypum and derived from the fleece of Greek sheep.

LAURAMIDE DEA is an alkanolamide used as a surfactant, foam booster and viscosity increasing agent.

LAURETH-7 is an alkoxylated alcohol, used as a surfactant.

LAURIC ACID is commonly found in vegetable fats, particularly coconut and laurel oil. The derivatives of lauric acid are widely used as a base in the production of soaps, detergents and lauryl alcohol because of their foaming and cleansing properties. This acid smells faintly similar to bay and produces plenty of large bubbles when added to soaps.

LAUROYL LYSINE is an amino acid derivative, used for its skin conditioning properties.

LAUROYL SARCOSINE – a mild surfactant used in shampoo and foam baths.

LAURYL ALCOHOL. A colourless, crystalline fatty alcohol used in chemical formulations for many purposes including to stabilise the emulsion, to increase the viscosity and as a skin conditioning material. It is derived from coconut oil and has a characteristic fatty odour.

LAURYL AMINOPROPYLGLYCINE is a substituted amino acid; a skin conditioning agent.

LAURYL BETAINE – a mild surfactant and skin conditioning material used in shampoo and foam baths.

LAURYL DIETHYLENEDIAMINOGLYCINE is a substituted amino acid; a skin conditioning agent and anti-static agent.

LECITHIN. Any of a group of phospholipids that are found in many living plants and animal tissues (especially egg yolks and soybeans), it is a natural emulsifier and stabiliser. Lecithin is also a natural antioxidant and skin conditioning material used in many cosmetics.

LIMNANTHES ALBA (meadowfoam oil). The winter annual wild flower called meadowfoam (*Limnanthes alba*) is native to the Pacific coast of North America, and it is from the seeds of this plant that the oil is derived. The oil is refined after extraction. When the oil is applied to the skin it is rapidly absorbed, leaving it soft and smooth.

LINOLEIC ACID (Vitamin F) is a fatty acid that occurs widely, in the form of glycerides, in vegetable fats and oils and in mammalian lipids. In cosmetics it is used as an emulsifier and to prevent dryness and roughness. Lack of linoleic acid results in symptoms similar to psoriasis and eczema. Together with arachidonic acid it is the most important essential fatty acid of the human diet.

LINOLENIC ACID is a fatty acid that occurs as a colourless liquid glyceride found in most oils. y-linolenic acid has been isolated from the seed oil of *Oenothera biennis*. This acid can act as an essential fatty acid. It is a skin conditioning and cleansing material.

LINUM USITATISSIMUM (linseed). An oil is derived

from dried ripe seeds of the herbaceous flax plant linseed *(Linum usitatissimum)*. An extract is also obtained from the seeds of the same plant. Linum Usitatissimum is a skin conditioning material used in shaving creams, medicated soaps and creams for its anti-inflammatory, healing properties.

LIPOSOMES, found in all living cells, are microscopic hollow sacs that are filled with moisturisers and other nourishing substances. They are formed from a variety of synthetic and natural water soluble substances, the phospholipids and lecithins among these being the most important. Liposomes act as carriers, transporting active substances easily into the skin because their compatibility with the skin's cellular membranes allows them to be easily accepted and metabolised. Some manufacturers claim that liposomes are able to penetrate easier into the skin to underlying layers when in a cream. They were originally developed as a method of introducing drugs into the body by by-passing destructive gut acid. Nanospheres are a more recent development.

LUCERNE. (See **MEDICAGO SATIVA**.)

LUFFA CYLINDRICA is the plant material derived from the fruit of this member of the gourd family, *Luffa cylindrica*. It is more commonly known as the loofah sponge, which is the dried skeleton of the fruit. (*Luffa cylindrica* is a synonym of *Luffa aegyptiaca*.) The dried particles swell up in the presence of water, giving the appearance of mini-sponges in formula. It makes a very gentle scrub base. (It is sometimes known by a trade name Lipo Luffa.)

MACADAMIA TERNIFOLIA NUT OIL. This fixed oil is obtained from the nuts of the Macadamia nut tree *(Macadamia ternifolia)* that is indigenous to the Brisbane area of Australia. The tree is now cultivated in other parts of Australia and the world, the largest producer of edible nuts being Hawaii. They also produce high quality Macadamia nut oil that is a good skin conditioning material used in cosmetics.

MAGNESIUM ALUMINIUM SILICATE is an inorganic salt used mainly for its absorbent, anti-caking properties.

MAGNESIUM ASCORBYL PHOSPHATE is a combination of organic salts used in cosmetic preparations as an antioxidant.

MAGNESIUM CARBONATE is an inorganic salt, used as a pH adjuster and adds bulk to skin care preparations.

MAGNESIUM STEARATE is a cosmetic colouring additive, which starts out as white but imparts colour when in solution. It is also used to add bulk to products.

MAGNESIUM SULPHATE is an inorganic salt, used to add bulk to cosmetic products.

MAIZE GLUTEN AMINO ACIDS are amino acids procured from a vegetable source and are said to be highly substantive and moisture retentive to skin.

MALIC ACID is found in many fruits and has a strong acidic taste. It is used as an antioxidant in skin care cosmetics and is present in hair lacquer. It has been known to cause irritation to the skin.

MALPIGHIA PUNICIFOLIA (acerola) is the extract obtained from the ripe fruit of the *Malpighia punicifolia* tree (more correctly known as *Malpighia glabra),* which is commonly known as acerola. The tree is native to tropical America. The extract is added to cosmetics for its claimed antioxidant properties, high content of Vitamin C and mineral salts which help to revitalise skin.

MANGANESE VIOLET is an inorganic salt and colour additive.

MANGIFERA INDICA (mango) is the EU-labelling name given to extracts obtained from the mango tree, *Mangifera indica.* An extract is derived from the mango fruit, and a fixed oil (mango seed oil) is derived from the kernels of the mango fruit *Mangifera indica.* Extracts are used in skin care products for their skin conditioning properties.

MANNITOL is a type of sugar alcohol known as a polyol. It is related to sorbitol, and is widely distributed in plants and fungi. It is obtained from natural sources and made synthetically. Mannitol is predominantly used in hand creams as a humectant and skin conditioning material.

MARANTA ARUNDINACEA (arrowroot). The rhizomes

of this white-flowered plant that originated in the West Indies and Central America, known as arrowroot (*Maranta arundinacea*), contain a starch that is extracted and crushed and added to moisturisers as an emollient factor.

MARIGOLD. (See **CALENDULA OFFICINALIS**.)

MARIS SAL (sea salt). This is the EU-labelling name given to the mixture of inorganic salts which originally come from natural sea water. It is used as a skin conditioning material.

MEDICAGO SATIVA (commonly known as alfalfa or lucerne) is extracted from the leguminous alfalfa plant, *Medicago sativa*. Although this plant is usually cultivated for animal feed, it serves as a commercial source of chlorophyll and carotene. For centuries there have been anecdotal reports that alfalfa leaves relieved kidney, bladder and prostate problems, and were supposedly used to relieve inflammation, diabetic conditions and ulcers. Alfalfa is high in vitamin and protein content. It is used widely in sun care products because its active constituents, including carotenes, are said to help prevent erythema (reddening of the skin). This lessens the inflammatory effects of sunburn.

MEL (honey) is the EU-labelling name given to the well-known sugary substance manufactured by the honey bee, *Apis mellifera*. It is a biological and skin conditioning material and a humectant.

MELALEUCA ALTERNIFOLIA (tea tree oil) is a fairly new ingredient on the market, and is obtained by steam distillation of the leaves of *Melaleuca alternifolia*. This shrubby tree originates from Australia and is now grown there in commercial plantations. Tea tree oil was first sold commercially in the 1920s for dental and surgical use and has become popular as it is reputed to contain non-irritating, germicidal properties that help relieve fungal and bacterial skin infections. Some cosmetic formulators use it in face creams as it is said to help increase the elasticity of the skin.

MENTHOL is obtained from the perennial herb peppermint and other species of mint oils (such as spearmint, pennyroyal, apple mint, etc.) for use mainly in creams, perfumes, aftershave lotions and skin fresheners. Menthol is unlikely to cause problems if used carefully and in moderation; the cool feeling it produces on the skin can turn to a burning sensation if used at too high concentrations.

METHICONE – a silicone derivative used as a skin conditioning agent.

METHYL CELLULOSE (also called cellulose, methyl ether) has the ability to swell in water and subsequently increase volume. It is processed from wood pulp or chemical cotton using alcohol. It is used in skin care preparations as an emulsion stabiliser and viscosity increasing agent.

METHYLCHLOROISOTHIAZOLINONE is an organic compound and powerful preservative.

METHYLISOTHIAZOLINONE is an organic compound and a preservative.

METHYLPARABEN. (See **PRESERVATIVES**.)

MEXICAN POPPY OIL (*Mbaruti* in Swahili) is extracted from *Argemone mexicana*, a plant that grows well in Tanzania as well as in other parts of the world. Its oil is used traditionally by Africans for treating dry skin conditions and other skin disorders. The fixed oil is used to enrich some modern skin care preparations.

MICA is a group of minerals consisting of certain silicates, which are found in certain types of rock. It consists of very thin sheets of mineral material that splits easily. In cosmetics it is used to add sparkle to a product.

MICROCRYSTALLINE WAX. (See **CERA MICRO-CRISTALLINA**.)

MINERAL OIL. (See **PARAFFINUM LIQUIDUM**.)

MINERAL SPIRITS. A complex combination of hydrocarbons obtained by the fractional distillation of petroleum.

MINERAL WAXES are derived from by-products of the petroleum industry. These waxes are commonly used as base ingredients in the cosmetics industry because they have different melting points. Ozokerite is a mixture of hydrocarbons originating from petroleum. When this brown or grey wax is refined, a hard white microcrystalline wax known as ceresin is produced.

MINERALS. Some minerals are incorporated into products for greasy skin care; sulphur is a favourite. However,
leading American dermatologist Professor Albert M Kligman
has made it known that, in his research, sulphur actually helps
to establish and increase comedones (blackheads). As blackheads are one of the least desirable effects of greasy skin, the
manufacturing of sulphur ointments and creams would be
best avoided.

MINK OIL. (See **MUSTELA**.)

MUCOPOLYSACCHARIDE. (See **GLYCOSAMINO-
GLYCAN**.)

MUD. *Mud, mud, glorious mud. There's nothing quite like
it for cooling the blood.* The cosmetic form of mud – a
mixture of a powder and a liquid – is used in facial masques.
Mud-packs are also popularly used. These, particularly those
from the Dead Sea, are said to be rich in minerals and salts
and contain healing and therapeutic properties.

MUSA SAPIENTUM (banana). Extractives and their
modified derivatives are obtained from the banana, *Musa
sapientum.* Banana extract is obtained from the banana fruit,
and banana leaf extract is obviously derived from the
banana's leaves. It is used for its emollient properties.

MUSK – the oily, strong-smelling substance taken from
the sexual glands of the male musk deer of central Asia – was
once used in perfumes for the sole purpose of attempting to
attract the opposite sex. The active constituent of musk,
muscone, is now made synthetically, but there is no duplication of natural musk.

MUSTELA (mink oil). This oil gained popularity supposedly after a mink farmer reported how soft his hands were
after handling the animals! Extractives from mink oil can be
used in emollients for soothing dry skin, but today it is not a
commonly used ingredient. This oil is a by-product of the
mink fur industry, extracted from the sub-dermal fatty tissues
of the animal. It used to be popular because it contains a
particular compound which makes it better than most vegetable oils when it comes to being absorbed by the skin and
leaving a soft non-oily feel upon it. It is also not prone to

rancidity. Synthetic mink is now produced and is more commonly used than the animal extract.

MYRISTIC ACID is a solid organic acid which is found naturally in butter acids particularly nutmeg butter, mace, lovage and coconut oils, and in most animal and vegetable fats. It is a surfactant and cleaning agent, when combined with potassium as myristic acid soap. It provides a generous lather and is used in shaving soaps, cleansers and creams.

MYRISTYL ALCOHOL is a fatty alcohol made of white crystals prepared from fatty acids. It is a skin conditioning material often used in handcreams and lotions and cold creams to give the product a soft velvety feel. It is also an emulsion stabiliser.

MYRISTYL MYRISTATE is an ester used as a skin conditioner.

NANOSPHERES. These are tiny, artificially manufactured micro-capsules, coated with gelatine, that trap moisturising agents, vitamins, plant extracts and an active ingredient and deliver them into the skin. Some cosmetic formulators claim that nanospheres can repair the skin as well as prevent further sun damage to it.

NEEM SEED OIL (**MELIA AZADIRACHTA**) is extracted from the seeds of the neem tree *Melia zazio-irachta*, which grows in India. The bark, roots, fruit and leaves are used by the Ayurvedic people for treating skin wounds and diseases, and for preventing gum disorders. Even twigs are used as toothbrushes or chewed since the plant's natural antiseptic properties help prevent pyorrhoea and tooth decay. Neem is also taken internally by some cultures to eliminate worms. The oil has a long history of safety. In skin care cosmetics it is used as a skin conditioning material.

NGALI NUT OIL is obtained from the Ngali nut tree (*Canarium indicum*) which is related to several other nut-bearing species of *Canarium*. The nuts from these trees are usually described as thick-shelled and difficult to crack. Ngali nut trees are widely distributed throughout the Solomon

Islands and occur in three species, the most common of which is the *Canarium indicum*. Cosmetic formulators use the oil for its emulsifying and emollient properties. It makes an ideal base for soaps and moisturising lotions.

NIACINAMIDE (Vitamin B3) is a compound used for its skin conditioning capabilities.

NIOSOMES are similar in structure to liposomes and are prepared from nonionic surfactants.

OCTOCRYLENE is an ester, and an ultra violet light absorber.

OCTYL COCOATE is an ester used as a skin conditioner and emollient.

OCTYL HYDROXYSTEARATE is an ester used as a skin conditioner and emollient.

OCTYL METHOXYCINNAMATE is a popular ultra violet light absorbing chemical used in many sun products. It is derived from balsam of Peru, cocoa leaves, cinnamon leaves and storax (trees or shrubs of tropical or sub-tropical regions). It is an ester and is soluble in oils but not in water.

OCTYL PALMITATE is an ester, used in cosmetics as a skin conditioning agent and emollient.

OCTYL STEARATE is an ester used as a skin conditioner and emollient.

OCTYLDODECANOL is a type of alcohol widely used as an emulsifier, an emollient with good spreading ability, a surfactant, a skin conditioning material and an opacifying agent.

OCTYLDODECYL STEAROYL STEARATE is an ester, used as a skin conditioner.

OENOTHERA BIENNIS is the EU-labelling name for an extract and an oil of the annual herb, evening primrose. The oil comes from the seeds of the *Oenothera biennis* herb. The oil contains a high proportion of y-linoleic acid (GLA) – a polyunsaturated fatty acid, which is chemically changed into hormones and prominent hormonal substances in body tissues called prostaglandin. This acid is extremely beneficial during times of premenstrual tension, high blood pressure and inflammation. It is also an excellent emollient. Evening primrose extract is derived from the roots and body of the annual herb.

OILS, FATS AND WAXES. Fatty raw materials are widely used in the cosmetics industry. These materials come from purified natural vegetable oils, land or sea animal oils, fats and waxes or petroleum oils and waxes. Synthetic derivatives are made from these natural sources.

Natural oils and fats are obtained from animals such as mink or ox (i.e. tallow), or from vegetable sources such as seeds like soya, sesame and sunflower, as well as from the fruit or seed of oil-bearing trees such as palm, avocado pear and olive. These natural oils and fats are produced in three main ways:

1. Mechanical pressing may be applied to plants by a screw press or hydraulic press employing heat, but only to those plants yielding 15-20 per cent oil. Cold-pressing is another method whereby the oil is squeezed from the plant material with no added heat, ensuring a pure, high quality oil as neither heat nor solvent disturbs the natural content. It is easier to cold-press materials such as olives and avocado pears, second best would be nuts; and seeds would be the hardest to cold-press.

2. Solvent (i.e. chemical) extraction dissolves out the oil. The part of the plants to be processed are ground, steam cooked and then mixed with the solvents (mostly from petroleum). The solvents then have to be completely eliminated.

3. Boiling in water. Animal fats are generally subjected to boiling as they are insoluble in water, form a layer on top which can be scooped off and purified, and they also have a solid or semi-solid texture at room temperature.

After extraction, it is common practice in large scale oil production to refine the oils and fats to remove impurities which may include moisture, free fatty acids, colourings, resins, gums and vitamins. The aim is to improve their colour, odour and chemical and physical stability. More than two thousand natural fats and oils are used in cosmetic formulation, each having slightly different properties. Mostly they provide moisture, emolliency, contain activators of skin metabolism and natural sun filters, plus they function as carriers of certain vitamins.

Natural waxes are obtained from vegetable and animal tissues by means of fusion or extraction with solvents and are thereafter refined and hydrogenated. They are used extensively in cosmetics as they enhance the appearance of the skin, although it is important they are decolourised and deodorised so that a standard material results.

Hydrocarbons used in cosmetics are by-products of the petroleum industries, for example, paraffin oils and paraffin wax, and these are sometimes known as mineral oils to differentiate between some other hydrocarbons obtained from animals and plants, for example, palm oil and shark liver oil.

Fatty acids. Most fatty acids come from animal and vegetable fats and oils by hydrolysis and purification.

Synthetics are generally obtained from vegetable materials such as coconut oil, or animal fats such as tallow, which are treated by hydrolysis or are hydrogenated.

OLEA EUROPAEA (olive oil). This is the fixed oil expressed from ripe olive fruits of the olive tree *Olea europaea* and made into emollients, soaps, products for ageing skin and massage oils. While using olive oil in cooking is said to be beneficial to one's health (due to its ability to balance cholesterol levels in the body and also to prevent arterial damage due to its antioxidant activity), in cosmetics it is also beneficial. Olive oil is used to soothe irritation and is an excellent internal and external lubricant.

OLEIC ACID is an oily, liquid, unsaturated acid occurring in a variety of animal and vegetable fats and oils. When exposed to air it can become rancid. It is used in cold creams, pre-shave lotions, toilet and soft soaps as a cleansing agent and surfactant.

OLEYL ACETATE is an ester used as a skin conditioner and emollient.

OLEYL ALCOHOL is used in cosmetics for manufacturing wetting agents and anti-foam agents, as well as in emollients. It is an unsaturated fatty alcohol found in most fish oils, and is oily to the touch. It can also be manufactured synthetically. For cosmetic use, oleyl alcohol is obtained by way of oleic acid or methyl oleate, from olive oil, tallow, palm oil or canola oil. It is a skin conditioning material.

OPUNTIA TUNA – prickly pear. (See **CACTUS EXTRACT**.)

ORANGE ROUGHY OIL. (See **HOPLOSTETHUS**.)

ORBIGNYA OLEIFERA (Babassu oil). A costly ingredient in some soaps, Babassu oil is extracted from the kernels of the Babassu palm *Orbignya oleifera* that grows in Brazil. One of the strongest features of this oil is that it scores low when tested for its comedo-producing potential, which is why it is used in creams for adolescents, designed to avoid a spotty skin.

ORCHIS MORIO is the name given to the extract taken from the flowers of the orchid *Orchis morio*. Commonly known as the green winged orchid, it grows wild in the south of England. 'Orchis' derives from the Greek word for testicle, which relates to the shape of the plant's tuber. An emollient is obtained from the tubers.

ORYZA SATIVA. This is the EU-labelling name given to various extracts from rice, *Oryza sativa*. Rice bran, rice bran extract, rice bran oil, rice extract, rice germ oil, rice starch and rice wax are all ingredients used in cosmetics and fall under the same labelling name. Rice bran oil is expressed from the broken coat of rice grain, which is rich in the fatty acids linoleic acid, Vitamins E and F, oleic acid, oryzanol and palmitic acid.

OVUM (egg). This is the EU-labelling name for a number of egg extracts that originate from whole fresh chicken eggs. Egg oil (here's egg on your face, literally: this oil is used as a facial moisturiser) is extracted from the yolks of eggs and is good for replenishing dehydrated skin. It replenishes by creating a film on the face, so allowing water to build up inside the tissues, making the skin tight initially and then soft. It also prevents friction when cosmetics containing it are rubbed on the skin. The oil is a combination of emollients and emulsifiers. Egg powder derives from the whole dried chicken egg, and is often used in creams, face masques and bath products. Egg yolk extract comes from the yolk of the egg only.

OYSTER NUT OIL. The oyster nut (*Kweme* in Swahili) is a huge perennial dioecious (having both male and female reproductive organs on separate plants) vine. It is indigenous to East and Central Africa and grows in forests. The nuts live within the tree's enormous gourd-like pods that can weigh up to 25kg each. The kernels are extracted from the seed by hand, then are washed and dried in the sun before being cold-pressed to extract the golden yellow oil. Traditionally, African women have used the oil to soften their skin and rub it into their breasts supposedly to improve their milk supply.

OZOKERITE is a hydrocarbon wax. In its crude state ozokerite is no longer easily procured. Instead, various hydrocarbons with properties similar to the original have been developed. These types of waxes help to form stable emulsions.

PALM KERNEL OIL. (See **ELAEIS GUINEENSIS**.)

PALMITIC ACID is a white crystalline solid saturated fatty acid, and is used as an emulsifying and cleansing material. It occurs naturally in plant oils and animal fats, and for cosmetic purposes is extracted from palm oil, Japan wax and Chinese vegetable tallow.

PANAX GINSENG EXTRACT (ginseng) comes from the roots of the perennial plant *Panax ginseng*. It helps to smooth and prevent dry skin, increase the skin's elasticity and to help restore a first-rate moisture level due to its vitamin and hormone content. Traditionally ginseng was used to soothe boils, sores and bruises, and is often used as an appetite stimulant and to alleviate coughs and chest disorders.

PANTHENOL – an alcohol. (See **VITAMINS**.)

PANTOTHENIC ACID. (See **VITAMINS**.)

PARABEN. (See **PRESERVATIVES**.)

PARAFFIN (paraffin waxes and hydrocarbon waxes). These waxes are a combination of hydrocarbons obtained from petroleum by distillation processes. They are translucent, odourless, tasteless and are not flexible but feel oily. When fully refined, the waxes are white. Paraffin is often used in cosmetics as a thickener and moisturiser, and is also used as a substitute for beeswax.

PARAFFINUM LIQUIDUM is the EU-labelling name for mineral oil. It is a liquid combination of a number of hydrocarbons originating from petroleum. It is refined considerably by acid treatment and hydrogenation, which gets rid of any unsaturated impurities. Technical names for this ingredient are: heavy mineral oil, liquid paraffin, paraffin oil, light mineral oil. Paraffinum liquidum is occlusive, easily emulsified, safe and inexpensive, and therefore used extensively in cosmetic formulation particularly as a skin conditioning material and emollient. As it lies on the skin's surface it is excellent for use in cleansers and also in massage products.

PARFUM is the EU-labelling name for perfume, which is basically a combination of alcohol and fragrant essential oils obtained from plants or made synthetically. *Parfum* is the French word for perfume. (See also Chapter 7.)

PASSIFLORA INCARNATA (passionflower). Passionflower extract is derived from the flowers of the passionflower, *Passiflora incarnata,* a climbing plant which grows wild in southern USA and is now cultivated in France. Passionflower oil is the fixed oil that is expressed from the seeds of *Passiflora incarnata.* The oil is used in skin care products designed for sensitive skin and in relaxing bath products because of its calming properties. And, just to confuse everybody, there is **PASSIFLORA EDULIS**, which is also a passionflower extract, fruit extract or oil, and is derived from *Passiflora edulis.* There are, indeed, other passionflowers that are used for cosmetic purposes.

PEGs. (For any item with the prefix PEG-, see **POLYETHYLENE GLYCOLS**.)

PENTAHYDROSQUALENE is a hydrocarbon, used as a skin conditioning agent.

PERFUME. (See **PARFUM**.)

PERSEA GRATISSIMA (avocado) is the EU-labelling name given to a number of extracts and derivatives from the avocado pear tree, *Persea gratissima.* Avocado extract derives from the avocado fruit; avocado leaf extract is obtained from the leaves of the same plant; avocado oil comes from crushing the dried flesh of another species of avocado pear, *Persea americana*. This fixed oil is made up of the glycerides of fatty acids and is a very emollient oil. Avocado oil contains Vitamins A, B and D and lecithin. It is used in cosmetics as a fatting agent and emollient. A wax is obtained by chilling the oil and filtering the resultant substance, which is used in emollients, shampoos and organic cosmetics. The oil is credited with soothing irritated skin and containing healing properties.

PETROLATUM (a technical name is petroleum jelly). Obtained from petroleum, this semi-transparent, semi-solid mixture of hydrocarbons is a gelatinous substance used as a base for many skin care creams for its skin conditioning properties. In its pure state it provides the skin with an oily film which prevents moisture evaporation from within. It is one of the least expensive and most effective skin protectors. However, it is difficult to remove from the skin and can cause comedones by clogging skin pores.

PHASEOLUS. Green bean (*Phaseolus lunatus*) extract and kidney bean (*Phaseolus vulgaris*) extract both come under the same name phaseolus for EU-labelling purposes. Green bean extract comes from the unripe beans of the *Phaseolus lunatus*. The oil extracted from the seeds of the kidney bean *Phaseolus vulgaris* is used mainly as a carrier. It helps to relieve pruritus and is particularly soothing on acned skin.

PHENOXYETHANOL is an aromatic ether alcohol which can be obtained from phenol. It is an oily liquid used as a preservative, fixative for perfume, insecticide, bacteriacide and as a topical antiseptic. It can also be used as a solvent for lotions, aftershaves, shampoos and skin creams.

PHENYL DIMETHICONE is a silicone polymer, used as a skin conditioning agent.

PHENYL TRIMETHICONE is of the chemical classes silicones and silanes, used as a skin conditioning agent.

PHYTOSTEROLS are plant fatty alcohols similar to human hormones but there is no evidence that they can act like the human ones. However, they are said to have an anti-inflammatory effect on the skin.

PLACENTAL ENZYMES, LIPIDS AND PROTEINS are all obtained from human and animal placentas. In cosmetics, these placental extracts are used predominantly for their vitamin and female hormone content and skin conditioning properties. They have been said to improve the appearance of ageing skin when added to a cosmetic by increasing the skin's oxygen absorption and encouraging cell metabolism, although others dispute this claim. In the EU the use of human placental derivatives has been banned.

PLANTAGO LANCEOLATA is an extract that is derived from the leaves of the plantain, *Plantago lanceolata*. This is the Eurasian perennial herb plantain (not the tropical banana-like plantain), that is found in much of Britain and Europe, in grasslands, roadsides, riverbanks, etc. It has lance-like, ribbed leaves and is commonly known as the ribwort plantain. Extracts from the plant are used as an emollient, demulcent and astringent.

PLASTICIZERS. These are chemical substances added to materials to soften and improve the flexibility of a material or substance without changing its chemical nature. For example, silicone glycols plasticise hair spray resins to stop them being too brittle.

POLLEN EXTRACT is a biological extract taken from flower pollen. It has a high content of proteins, vitamins, minerals and amino acids.

POLOXAMER 184 is a polymeric ether used as a surfactant and cleanser.

POLYETHYLENE (another name for polythene) is derived from petroleum gas or by dehydrating alcohol. Polyethylene is one of a group of thermoplastics that is resistant to chemicals, has a low moisture absorption rate and good insulating properties. It is usually used in cosmetics as granules for a scrub.

POLYETHYLENE DILAURATE is a mild surfactant often used in baby oils.

POLYETHYLENE GLYCOLS (**PEGs**) are synthetic

materials incorporated into a formulation to ensure that the required viscosity, humectancy and melting point are obtained. They are present in many cosmetics, notably cream bases and pharmaceutical ointments. They are formed by adding ethylene oxide to ethylene glycol. PEG is the abbreviation used for polyethylene glycol. Should a PEG be listed together with another ingredient (e.g. **PEG-8 stearate**), it means that a polyethylene glycol (PEG) chain has been added to the ingredient to enhance water solubility. The numbers that come after PEG on a label indicate the chain length of the PEG. (For example, PEG-8 stearate will have a chain length of eight units.) The bigger the figure, the more likely the polymer is to be viscous or a semi/solid e.g. PEG-400 is a liquid; PEG-4000 is a powder. All PEG-stearates are emulsifying agents that are used in different quantities in different types of products.

PEG-4 ISOSTEARATE; PEG-8 ISOSTEARATE; PEG-10 ISOSTEARATE are all alkoxylated carboxylic acid, used in skin care preparations as emulsifying agents.

PEG-6 STEARATE is most often used as an emulsifier in the manufacture of cleansing products.

PEG-8. This is used to regulate the moisture and consistency of some lotions, shaving products and hair care products.

PEG-8 DISTEARATE. This is the polyethylene glycol diester of stearic acid. It is used in cosmetics as an emulsifying agent.

PEG-8 STEARATE – an emulsifier and thickening agent often used in creams, moisturising products and hair care products.

PEG-32 STEARATE – most commonly used in moisturisers and face products as a cleansing and solubilizing agent.

PEG-100 STEARATE – a stabiliser and emulsifier for creams and lotions. It is also incorporated into hair care products, toiletries and some perfumes.

PEG-150. This refers to long polymers of ethylene oxide, usually in the form of a waxy compound.

POLYGLYCERYL-2 CAPRATE is basically a glyceryl

ester and derivatives of it. Used for its emulsifying and emollient properties.

POLYISOBUTENE is a synthetic hydrocarbon polymer used as a cosmetic binder, film former and viscosity-increasing agent.

POLYMETHYL METHACRYLATE is a synthetic polymer used for its film forming abilities.

POLYOXYETHYLENE COMPOUNDS and derivatives are generally liquids of a waxy or oily consistency, used as emulsifiers in creams and lotions.

POLYQUATERNIUM-39. A polyquaternium is known in the industry as QUATS – quaternary ammonium compounds – which are basically synthetic polymers. It is used as a film former.

POLYSORBATES are widely used as stabilisers and emulsifiers in various cosmetic products.

POTASSIUM ALUM (i.e. alum) is an inorganic salt used in astringents and aftershave lotions as a styptic and was once used to help prevent aluminium chloride from causing skin irritation in antiperspirants. However, aluminium chloride is no longer used in antiperspirants on general sale because it was found to irritate the skin – it also corroded the cans! Technical names for this ingredient, commonly known as alum, are often used on product labels. These include Aluminium Potassium Sulphate; Alum, Potassium; and Potassium Aluminium Sulphate.

POTASSIUM CETYL PHOSPHATE is a combination of esters of phosphoric acid and cetyl alcohol. It is used in cosmetics as an emulsifying agent.

POTASSIUM HYDROXIDE (also known as caustic potash) is prepared for cosmetic use by electrolysis of potassium chloride. It saponifies fats, and is often the counter ion to the fatty acid of liquid soaps. It is highly corrosive so is never used on the skin entirely by itself.

POTASSIUM SORBATE is an organic salt and used as a preservative.

PPG is the short term for polypropylene glycol.

PPG-2 METHYL ETHER is an alkoxylated alcohol, used as a solvent.

PPG-15 STEARYL ETHER is an alkoxylated alcohol, used as a skin conditioning agent.

PRESERVATIVES are incorporated into cosmetics and toiletries to protect the products from contamination by micro-organisms. These substances are strictly controlled. There are lists as to what can be used and at what levels. All on the positive list are synthetic. Ideally, a preservative should have antibacterial and antifungal properties, it should not be toxic nor contain irritants, and it should have the ability to be added to other products without causing change or any adverse effects. The **paraben** group of preservatives is widely used because of its anti-microbial properties and high safety level. **Butylparaben** is more effective in the acid pH range. Most often it is used in combination with other preservatives to increase the range of preservative activity. **Methylparaben** is most popularly used because of its low sensitizing potential. It has been used for many years to fight mould and bacteria, as has **propylparaben** – also one of the most widely used preservatives because of its low toxicity. **Quaternary ammonium compounds** are also widely used in cosmetics. These compounds are preservatives, antiseptics, surfactants and germicides. One of the most widely utilised antibacteria preservatives is **Imidazolidinyl Urea**, popular with cosmetic formulators because of its low potential to cause allergic reactions. It is not used on its own but rather in conjunction with parabens. **Bronopol** is another preservative still being used mainly for wash-off products. It is effective against many micro-organisms but particularly against fungi and yeast. In small concentrations (i.e. 0.01-0.1 per cent) it is generally non-toxic to humans. The full chemical name for this ingredient is **2-bromo-2 nitropropane-1,3-diol**, which is sometimes used on labels. **Formaldehyde** is a volatile aldehyde, a colourless, poisonous, highly irritating gas with a pungent odour. In cosmetics it serves as a cheap but effective preservative as well as being a germicide, disinfectant and fungicide. It is found in shower and bath products, is commonly used in the detergent industry and for preserving natural extracts. Formaldehyde is formed by methyl alcohol being oxidised and mixed with water. Allergic skin reactions to this preservative have occurred. **Quaternium 15** is an all-purpose preservative, effective against yeast, bacteria and mould. However, in leave-on cosmetics, irritation such as dermatitis has occurred in certain individuals. This was due to the release of formaldehyde; however, the latest types of quaternium 15 have most likely been made in such a manner so that formaldehyde release does not occur. **Sodium benzoate** consists of white odourless crystals or powder and is used as antiseptics and preservatives in eye creams and vanishing creams.

Maurene writes: A company keen to promote its latest preservative once sent me a 25ml sample. The accompanying data sheet did not inspire me since the product in its raw state seemed detrimental to skin and eyes and if ingested. Four weeks before this I had bought a delightful Rhodesian ridgeback puppy named Sula. One Saturday, by some feat, Sula managed to climb onto the work-bench where the preservative lay. That evening I found the chewed remains of the container minus contents. In near panic I was convinced I'd murdered her. Without the necessary toxicological data the vet was powerless to help and we had to sweat it out until the Monday morning when I could extract information from the company's technical department. A chemist from there said, rather drily: 'Don't bury Sula.' God preserve us. (Sula was quite unaffected!)

PROPOLIS CERA (**propolis**) is a greenish brown resinous aromatic substance collected by bees from trees, flowers, shrubs and other plants for use in constructing hives. It is a component of beeswax, commonly known as bee glue or hive dross. The bees use it to seal any cracks in the hive and, as it is an excellent antiseptic, they also use it to wrap up any invading predators. People used it centuries ago for soothing irritated skin, and now it is still used for its healing, cleansing and sun protecting properties, but it can cause allergies.

PROPYLENE GLYCOL is a compound usually found in anti-freeze and brake fluid, but in cosmetics it is the most commonly used moisture-bearing substance apart from water.

It is used as a humectant, a wetting agent and a solvent in many cosmetic products. However, it can cause irritation to some skins when used in high concentrations. and researchers are looking to replace it with safer glycols such as poly-ethylene glycol and butylene glycol.

PROPYLENE GLYCOL LAURATE is an ester used for its emollient and emulsifying properties.

PROPYLPARABEN. (See **PRESERVATIVES**.)

PRO-VITAMIN B5 is the precursor to Vitamin B5 (that is, it forms Vitamin B5 in-situ).

PRUNUS AMYGDALUS AMARA (bitter almond oil). A volatile essential oil is extracted from the kernels of the bitter almond tree, *Prunus amygdalus amara*. The tree is widely cultivated in Italy, Spain, France, the USA and Australia. Bitter almond essential oil is obtained by macerating and then distilling the ripe kernels for scenting and flavouring pur-poses. This refining process removes dihydrocyanic acid or prussic acid, the extremely poisonous aqueous solution of hydrogen cyanide. Among its ingredients are benzaldehyde and hydrogen cyanide. **PRUNUS AMARA** is the EU-labelling name given to bitter almond extract, which is derived from the seeds of the almond tree *Prunus amygdalus amara*.

PRUNUS ARMENIACA (apricot) is the EU name given to a number of extracts of the apricot, *Prunus armeniaca*. Apricot extract is taken from the fruit, apricot kernel extract is derived from the kernels of the apricot, and a fixed oil (apricot kernel oil) is obtained from the cold-pressing of the kernels of varieties of *Prunus armeniaca*. The oil can contain impurities (cynoglycosides) when unrefined. Used mainly as a carrier, this oil has good moisturising properties and contains a high percentage of Vitamin E. It is absorbed rapidly by the skin and helps retain the skin's elasticity. Apricot leaf extract is derived from the leaves of the tree, and apricot seed powder is the resultant powder when the apricot's seeds are crushed.

PRUNUS AVIUM is the EU-labelling name given to the extract and pit oil extracted from the sweet cherry, *Prunus* *avium*. It is grown in many parts of the world including Europe, Asia, Australia, the USA and South America. The extract is used by some cosmetic formulators in astringents for revitalising purposes.

PRUNUS CERASUS (bitter cherry extract). The bitter cherry extract has a high fatty acid content, which is of particular interest to formulators of skin care emulsions. It is extracted from the kernels or pits of the sour or pie cherry *Prunus cerasus*.

PRUNUS DULCIS (sweet almond) is the EU-labelling name given to a number of extracts of the fruit and seeds of the sweet almond tree, *Prunus amygdalus dulcis*. Sweet almond oil is the fixed oil obtained from cold-pressing the kernels of sweet almonds and is a favourite in massage and skin care cosmetics for its emollient properties. Other extracts from the same species include sweet almond meal, which is what remains when the oil is taken from the almond's dried ripe seeds, sweet almond extract (taken from the fruit), and sweet almond seed extract, which derives from its dried ripe seeds.

PRUNUS PERSICA (peach) is the EU-labelling name given to a number of extracts of the peach, *Prunus persica*. An oil is expressed from the kernel of the peach fruit. It is used as an oil base in emollients and has a smell similar to that of the almond. Other extracts include peach juice (expressed from the flesh of the peach) and peach leaf extract (derived from the peach tree's leaves).

PUMICE is a light porous volcanic rock. In cosmetics it is used as an abrasive powder in skin cleansing grains and soaps designed for acne sufferers and for hand cleansing preparations. If applied daily to dry, sensitive skin it will cause irritation, but only due to the constant friction. People use the complete stone to remove dead or rough skin particularly on the feet.

PVP is short for **POLYVINYLPYRROLIDONE**. It is a solid synthetic resin resembling albumen which is used in the cosmetic, food and medical industries. In cosmetics it is used in products such as waterproof sunscreens and lipsticks to ensure water and wear resistance.

QUATERNARY AMMONIUM COMPOUNDS. (See **PRESERVATIVES**.)

QUATERNIUM 15. (See **PRESERVATIVES**.)

RETINYL PALMITATE (also known as **Vitamin A palmitate**) is the ester of retinol and palmitic acid. It is a skin conditioning material and an antioxidant, which maintains skin softness by acting as an anti-keratinising agent and improving its water barrier properties.

RHUS SUCCEDANEA (Japan wax). Japan wax is vegetable fat derived from the flesh of the fruit of the *Rhus succedanea* berries. In cosmetics it is used as a binder and viscosity increasing material. The wax imparts good feel to the skin.

RIBES NIGRUM is the fixed oil extracted from high quality blackcurrant seeds of the blackcurrant plant, *Ribes nigrum*. The seeds are neutralised to reduce acidity and bleached under vacuum, ensuring the oil is free of impurities. Tests have shown that after applying an emulsion containing blackcurrant seed oil to human skin there was a noticeable increase in the linoeic and linolenic acid content and a significant improvement in dry skin. (Linoleic acid, a-linolenic and y-linolenic acid or GLA, also known as essential fatty acids or Vitamin F, cannot be synthesized by the body but are vital for its proper functioning, in particular, the skin.) Blackcurrant oil is rich in this GLA (full term for it is gamma linolenic acid), the same amount as that found in evening primrose oil and borage. In cosmetics it is used for its skin conditioning and emollient properties. An extract deriving from the fruit of the same plant is also used in cosmetics.

RICINOLEIC ACID is a fatty extract from castor bean seeds that contains large quantities of this acid. It is a cleansing material used in soaps and contraceptive jellies, and as a matter of interest, it is this acid which is considered responsible for the laxative properties of castor oil.

RICINUS COMMUNIS (castor oil). This is the fixed oil that comes from the pressed castor bean seeds of a perennial plant native to Africa, namely *Ricinus communis*. It is now cultivated widely in most tropical countries for commercial purposes including for cosmetics. Beans of the castor oil plant contain ricin, a highly toxic chemical, although refined castor oil itself is free from this nasty substance. Consuming just a few seeds has caused death in adults, cattle and in poultry. In Africa, mixing castor oil seeds with food is a well-known means of infanticide, and the oil is used to poison cockroaches. In Egypt the plant is grown around houses to repel mosquitoes. It is a constituent of embalming fluids and imparts emollient and lubricative properties to many cosmetic preparations. Castor oil has been used in folk medicine for centuries. It is popularly used by cosmetic formulators as it is a good vehicle for dispersing colours in lipsticks and other cosmetics.

ROSA CENTIFOLIA is the EU-labelling name for a number of extracts and derivatives of the cabbage rose, *Rosa centifolia*. An oil and an extract are used in cosmetics, mainly for scenting purposes. An extract is water, which is the liquid that is collected from the scent carrying parts of the cabbage rose's flowers (though this is not how rose water is made – see below).

ROSE WATER is the scented water produced when rose petals are distilled in water or steam. Often it is combined with glycerine. It has soothing, cooling and cleansing properties, and is found in many cosmetic preparations for these reasons as well as to scent the product delicately.

ROSEHIP OIL is extracted from the seeds of the wild rose grown in China. Rich in Vitamin C, it is added to skin care cosmetics for its supposed antiseptic properties and for the fact that it leaves a lovely smooth feel to the skin.

ROYAL JELLY is food of the queen bee. It is a secretion from the pharyngeal glands of certain worker bees, produced for the sole purpose of nourishing the larvae, and particularly those larvae destined to become queen bees. It is a natural source of pantothenic acid and also contains essential minerals, fats, carbohydrates, water and Vitamins E and F. (See also **CERA ALBA**.)

SALICYLIC ACID. This antiseptic, fungicidal preservative is manufactured synthetically. Its main use in the cosmetics field is as a keratolytic agent in acne creams (it opens up the crusty surface of the comedo to allow the antiseptic in). It is also a denaturant and skin conditioning material, and is used in the treatment of conditions such as itching. It is a main component of aspirin. Natural forms of salicylic acid were once extracted from different plants including from the leaves of wintergreen shrubs and from bark of willow trees and sweet birch.

SALVIA HISPANICA (technical name is Chia oil) is the oil extracted from the crushed seeds of *Salvia hispanica*, a variety of sage. It is high in linoleic acid.

SAPONARIA OFFICINALIS EXTRACT (soapwort). The boiled extract of this perennial herb has been used by many a great-great-grandmother to work into a lather upon 'delicate hair' in an effort to strengthen it. Today, extract from the roots and leaves of soapwort *(Saponaria officinalis)* is used to relieve itchy skin and is added to skin cleansing products for its saponin (a constituent of specific plants with a steroid structure that foams when shaken) content. *Interestingly, soapwort was grown on the nineteenth century farms of the American Shakers, a sect founded in 1747 as an offshoot of the Quakers. Their quirk was to shake ecstatically; among other things they practised common ownership of property, farming and craftsmanship. Their shaking had no connection whatsoever with making soapwort foam – they simply did so in moments of religious ecstasy. Soapwort was grown for its curative powers on eczema, acne and venereal diseases, for its soothing effect on poison ivy rashes and its ability to eliminate toxins from the liver.*

SAPONIN. Any of a group of plant glycosides which foam when shaken in water. They are used for their detergent, foaming and emulsifying abilities in shaving creams, bath oils and shampoos. They are extracted from many plants including soapwort and sarsaparilla.

SEA SALT. (See **MARIS SAL**.)

SEAWEED contains an abundance of mineral salts including iodine, potassium, iron and calcium, as well as many vitamins, amino acids and alginates. It is also reputed to contain natural antibiotics which can heal minor infections. Certain green seaweed, as well as algae, have great potential for formulators of cosmetics, and research on them is currently being carried out. More than 17,000 species of red, green, blue and brown seaweed exist, but those currently used in cosmetics are extracted from the red and brown seaweed (see **CHONDRUS CRISPUS** and **ALGIN**). The thallus (the undifferentiated part) of seaweed is used, with a total of from 2 to 7 per cent being added to cosmetic formulations. Fresh seaweed is commonly used in the face masques that peel off in one piece. These types of masques prevent moisture from escaping through the skin, leaving the skin soft and moist.

SERICA (silk powder) is a finely crushed biological material obtained from the secretion of silkworm, the larva of the Chinese moth *Bombyx mori* that eats mulberry tree leaves (see **BOMBYX**). It is used in face powder predominantly for its ability to prevent cracking, aid humectancy and oil absorption.

SERINE is an amino acid, a skin conditioner.

SERUM ALBUMIN. Derived from cows' blood plasma, this substance carries essential fatty acids to the cells of the epidermis. When this serum and the essential fatty acids are placed on the skin it is reported to help the rate of cell renewal within the epidermis.

SESAMUM INDICUM (sesame). This is the EU-labelling name given to various extracts of the intensively cultivated East Indian tropical herbaceous plant, sesame (*Sesamum indicum*), which produces a rose-coloured or white flower. The crushed sesame seeds yield pale yellow, odourless sesame oil, which is used in the food industry as well as in skin care cosmetics as a skin softener and as a perfume fixative. The white and black varieties are the most cultivated in India, and, although the most favoured oil comes from the white seeds, the black seeds have the higher oil yield. Virgin oil is obtained by cold-pressing non-roasted seeds, which preserves its qualities. It is resistant to oxidation and is the most stable oil used in the manufacture of pharmaceuticals. Sesame extract and sesame seed are other extracts also derived from the seeds.

SHELLAC is the yellowish solid resinous substance secreted by the insect *Laccifer (Tachardia) lacca* (commonly known as the lac insect) which thrives on certain trees found in India and Thailand. The female insects deposit the resinous matter, which includes eggs and a viscous covering, on the branches. The species of the host tree, as well as the strain of the insect, determine the final colour and properties of the shellac to be processed for marketing. Twice a year this resin is harvested and then processed. It is refined for use in cosmetics by the solvent extraction process, where it is generally used as a binder and in the manufacture of mascara, hair conditioners and hair sprays. Most of the old 78 rpm records were made of shellac. The EU-labelling name for the ingredient used in cosmetics is **SHELLAC CERA** (a wax).

SILICA is an inorganic oxide occurring naturally as quartz. It is found in many rocks. When it is dried and heated in a vacuum, granules of white powder result and this is used in the cosmetics industry as an abrasive and an absorbent material, particularly in suntan gels and foot powders. Also used as an anti-caking and opacifying ingredient.

SILICA SILYLATE comes from the chemical class silicones and silanes, and is used as a skin conditioning agent and emollient.

SILICEOUS EARTH is purified silica often used in face masques. It is extracted through boiling with diluted acid which is then washed through a filter.

SILICON is a brittle metalloid element obtained from sand, clay, granite, felspar and quartz. It is usually a grey crystalline solid but it can also come in the form of a brown powder. Silicones are silicon derivatives.

SILICONE FLUID derives from silica found in rocks and sand. An extremely versatile emollient, it is used widely in the cosmetic field.

SILICONES are made from silicon. They are technically polymeric molecules (can be of a very high molecular weight or long chain) with a common backbone of silicon-oxygen linkages. Silicones can be described as any of a large class of compounds derived of silicon that are resistant to temperature, water and chemicals, and contain insulating and lubricating properties. They are therefore widely used as oils, water repellents, resins and rubbers. They can be found in hand lotions, protective creams, aftershave lotions and other cosmetic products.

SILK POWDER. (See **SERICA**.)

SILK WORM EXTRACT. (See **BOMBYX**.)

SIMETHICONE. A silicone oil and anti-foam compound which is used as a base ingredient in ointments. It protects the skin and is a medium for topical drugs.

SKATOLE is a potent-smelling, yellowish, fatty secretion that comes from the perineal glands of the civet, a spotted cat-like mammal of Africa and south Asia. Perfume manufacturers used it as an aromatic additive to enhance expensive floral perfumes. It was once widely used as a fixative in the manufacture of perfumes, but cosmetic formulators today more commonly use equally good and cheaper synthetic substitutes.

SODIUM ACETATE – an organic salt, used as a buffering agent.

SODIUM BENZOATE. (See **PRESERVATIVES**.)

SODIUM BICARBONATE (bicarbonate of soda and baking soda are frequently used technical names). This organic salt, commonly used in baking and medicinally for burns, is also used in cosmetics as an abrasive, a buffering material and pH adjuster. It is added to products designed to soothe skin, as well as in effervescent bath salts, toothpaste and mouthwashes. It can absorb odours and is used in deodorants. It has been known to cause irritation on very dry skin.

SODIUM BORATE (borax) is an inorganic salt and component of a modern cold cream. It is used as a pH adjuster. It is now known to be one of the components used by the Greek physician Galen who made the first cold cream.

SODIUM CARBOMER. An organic salt used to stabilise emulsions. It is also a film former and viscosity increasing agent.

SODIUM CARBONATE (soda ash is a common technical

name). A colourless or white odourless soluble inorganic salt found in ores situated in lake brines or seawater, sodium carbonate is a pH adjuster used in soaps, foot products, bath salts and vaginal douches.

SODIUM CETEARYL SULPHATE is the sodium salt of a combination of the sulphuric acid esters of cetyl and stearyl alcohol. It is a surfactant, used as a cleansing agent as well as an oil-in-water emulsifier for creams.

SODIUM CETYL SULPHATE is a surface active agent which is the sulphate ester of the alcohol. It is used mainly in the dye, soap and detergent industries, as well as medicinally. Sodium cetyl sulphate is marketed in the form of a paste.

SODIUM CHLORIDE. This is the common salt we put on our food (or are warned not to, as the case may be). It is an inorganic salt, widely used in cosmetics as a viscosity-increasing agent.

SODIUM CITRATE – an organic salt, used as a pH adjuster and buffering agent.

SODIUM COCOATE is the sodium salt of coconut acid which comes from the coconut. It is found in soaps as a surfactant, and cleansing and emulsifying agent.

SODIUM DEHYDROACETATE – an organic salt used as a preservative.

SODIUM DIHYDROXYETHYLGLYCINATE – a chelating agent.

SODIUM HYDROXIDE (commonly known as caustic soda) is a strongly alkaline solid used in the manufacture of soaps and as a pH adjuster and denaturant.

SODIUM LACTATE is the sodium salt of lactic acid and is a safe and inexpensive natural humectant, moisturiser and conditioner. It keeps a product's pH from becoming too acidic. It is a component of the stratum corneum of the skin but does not affect the pliability of the skin, unlike lactic acid.

SODIUM LAURETH SULPHATE is a surfactant. It is used in many products – shampoos, bath foam, liquid soap, etc.

SODIUM LAURYL SULPHATE is the sodium salt of lauryl sulphate. It is a surfactant and cleansing agent, popularly used by manufacturers of cleansers and soaps packaged with pump dispensers. It is used in some liquid soaps, cream depilatories and toothpastes.

SODIUM PALMITATE is a soap – technically, it is the sodium salt of palmitic acid. It is used as a surfactant, cleansing and emulsifying agent, and a viscosity-increasing agent.

SODIUM PCA – an organic salt used as a humectant and skin conditioner.

SODIUM POLYACRYLATE – the sodium salt of a synthetic polymer used as a viscosity increasing material.

SODIUM SESQUICARBONATE is an inorganic salt and pH adjuster, a mix of sodium bicarbonate and sodium carbonate. It is often added to bath salts to make them alkaline. High concentrations of it in products have been known to cause inflammed or itchy conditions in those with sensitive skins.

SODIUM STEARATE is the sodium salt of stearic acid. It is used as a cleansing agent and viscosity increasing material in stick perfumes, deodorant sticks, shaving lathers, soapless shampoos and as a waterproofing agent in various products.

SODIUM TALLOWATE is the sodium salt of tallow acid and is basically a soap. It is used as a surfactant, cleansing agent and foam booster and a viscosity-increasing agent.

SORBIC ACID is a carboxylic acid, in nature found in berries of the rowan or mountain ash *Sorbus aucuparia,* native to Britain and northern Europe but common in streets, gardens and parks everywhere. It is used as a preservative. Synthetic sorbic acid is also available for use in cosmetics.

SORBITAN OLEATE is derived from natural fats and oils for use in cosmetics as an emulsifier and mild cleansing and foaming agent. Most commonly it is found in soaps.

SORBITAN SESQUIOLEATE is a fatty ester derived from sorbitol, a white crystalline alcohol found in fruits such as rose hips and rowan berries, and is manufactured by the catalytic reduction of glucose with hydrogen. In cosmetics it is used as a surfactant and emulsifying agent.

SORBITAN STEARATE is made by reacting edible commercial stearic acid with sorbitol. It is a secondary emulsifier that helps formulate glossy emulsions.

SORBITOL for use in cosmetics is a humectant which can be used instead of glycerine in creams, ointments, masques, deodorants, hand lotions and anti-perspirants. As a humectant it draws moisture from the air into the skin; however, if the moisture content of the skin is greater than the air outside, it will actually draw moisture out of the skin. Sorbitol is present in most berries (such as the rowan) as well as in apples, pears, cherries, seaweed and algae.

SPLEEN EXTRACT. This biological additive is usually obtained from the spleen of cows and is added to skin care products as it is said to give the user a smoother skin.

SQUALENE is obtained from shark liver oil or other natural oils by hydrogenation. It also occurs in smaller quantities in plants such as olives, wheat germ and rice bran. It is used in cosmetics as a moisturiser and lubricant, and is also a perfume fixative.

SQUALI IECUR. The official EU-labelling name for shark liver oil, which is derived from the fresh livers of various species of shark but most commonly the sharks *Galeorhinus zyopterus* (commonly known as the Soup Fin Shark) and *Hypoprion brevirostris*. The oil is high in Vitamin A, which is why it is used in cosmetics.

STEARETH 20. An emulsifier in oil-in-water cosmetic formulations. The number indicates the degree of liquidity so that the higher the number, the more solid it is.

STEARIC ACID is an emulsifier and thickening agent that occurs naturally in many animal and vegetable fats including butter acids, tallow and cascarilla bark. Stearic acid, partly neutralised with alkalis or triethanolamine, is used in the preparation of emulsions. Its main use is as the primary emulsifier in a wide variety of creams and lotions. Stearic acid is the main ingredient of soap bars – this is usually present as the sodium of potassium soap. It gives pearliness to hand creams.

STEARYL ALCOHOL. Insoluble in water, it is a simple

fatty alcohol soluble in alcohol and ether. It is usually prepared from tallow or vegetable oil, commonly palm oil. Sometimes it is used instead of cetyl alcohol because of its softer nature at room temperature. It is an emulsion stabiliser, emulsifying agent and skin conditioning agent.

STEARYL CAPRYLATE is an ester, used as a skin conditioner.

STEARYL HEPTANOATE. An ester, used as a skin conditioner.

SUCROSE COCOATE is the ester of coconut acid and sucrose, which is used in cosmetics as a skin conditioner.

SULPHUR is a naturally occurring element used as a skin conditioning agent. (See also **MINERALS**.)

SUNFLOWER OIL. (See **HELIANTHUS ANNUUS**.)

SUPEROXIDE DISMUTASE is one of the most recent arrivals on the cosmetic scene used to combat the ageing process. It is an enzyme that strengthens the body against free radical damage (free radicals are destructive molecules that destroy healthy cells and so speed up the ageing process). It is found in aerobic cells.

SYMPHYTUM OFFICINALE (comfrey) is the EU-labelling name for extracts of the perennial comfrey herb, *Symphytum officinale*. An extract is taken from the roots and rhizomes of the herb, and a leaf extract and leaf powder derive from the leaves of the comfrey. The herb is well known for its healing of skin conditions.

TALC is such a soft mineral that it easily becomes a powder, and consists primarily of magnesium silicate, although it sometimes has a trace of aluminium silicate. It is an absorbent material, used also for anti-caking and as an opacifying ingredient.

TALLOW (**ADEPS BOVIS**). Obtained from the fatty tissue of cattle and sheep for manufacturing soap. It is also used in shaving cream, shampoo and lipstick production.

TALLOW GLYCERIDES. A combination of triglycerides (fats for consistency regulation for creams, lotions and make-up) derived from tallow. Used as emulsifying agents and surfactants. (See **TALLOW**.)

TARTARIC ACID is an organic acid found in many fruits. It is a pH adjuster, and its acid properties make it suitable for the production of bath salts.

TEA. (See **TRIETHANOLAMINE**.)

TEA-LACTATE. An amine salt, this is used as a skin conditioning agent.

TEA-LAURYL SULPHATE. This surfactant and emulsifier is used in bubble baths and various creams. Because of its degreasing properties it can cause the skin to dry out. It is a fairly mild surfactant but, as with all detergents, can irritate the skin to some extent.

TEREPHTHALYDIENE DICAMPHOR SULPHONIC ACID. This organic compound is used as an ultra violet light absorber.

TETRASODIUM EDTA (EDTA = ethylene diamine tetra acetic acid) is a powdered sodium salt that combines with metals. In cosmetics it is used as a preservative and as a sequestering and chelating agent.

THEOBROMA CACAO (cocoa). This is the EU-labelling name given to derivatives of the cocoa plant. Cocoa butter is the yellowish white fat obtained from the roasted seeds of the cocoa bean, *Theobroma cacao*. It is one of the most widely used ingredients in cosmetology as it is a natural emollient that softens and lubricates the skin. It is also often added to massage creams. The fat melts at body temperature but is brittle below 25°C. An extract also derives from this cocoa plant.

THYMUS EXTRACT is taken from the thymus gland of animals for use in skin creams. This organ produces cells which help the body's immune system fight invaders. Some cosmetic scientists say it is beneficial for improving cell functioning, while others disagree, suggesting the idea is purely a marketing ploy because very little gets into the skin cream itself.

TITANIUM DIOXIDE is an inorganic oxide that comes in the form of a white powder. It is used chiefly in colour cosmetics, but it is also an opacifying agent and a non-chemical SPF used in sunscreens. When it is applied, titanium dioxide sits on the skin's surface and disperses UV light. It comes in differing particle sizes, generally referred to as 'micro' or 'ultra'. The larger the particles, the more whiteness is left on the skin (see also **COLOURS**).

TOCOPHEROL (a technical name for it is Vitamin E) is a natural antioxidant obtained from edible vegetable oils. In the body it helps form normal red blood cells, muscle and other tissue. In skin care products tocopherol is used as an antioxidant, for stabilising essential oils and mineral oils, and to stabilise Vitamin A. Tocopherol helps to prevent general skin damage, it moisturises dry skin and improves its elasticity. (See **VITAMINS**.) It is used in many cosmetics, particularly in creams and lotions designed for older skins.

TOCOPHERYL ACETATE. This is an antioxidant that helps to prevent rancidity in unsaturated oils and sebum. It is the ester of tocopherol and acetic acid.

TRACE ELEMENTS (also known as micronutrients or oligo-elements) are any of a number of chemical elements such as iron, copper, zinc and magnesium that are present in plants and animals in very small amounts but are essential for the organism's life. In cosmetics they have a moisturisation value.

TRIBEHENIN is a fatty substance used for skin conditioning purposes.

TRICLOCARBANAMIDE – used as a cosmetic biocide.

TRICLOSAN is a phenol, used in deodorant. It is also a cosmetic biocide and preservative.

TRIETHANOLAMINE (**TEA** is the abbreviation) is a colourless fluid derived from ammonia and is used chiefly to form its salts with fatty acids such as stearic acid and oleic acids. Equal proportions of base and fatty acid form a soap that may be used as an emulsifying agent to produce fine-grained stable emulsions of the oil-in-water type.

TRIETHANOLAMINE STEARATE is used in making emulsions. It is the soap from triethanolamine and stearic acid, absorbs moisture and is found in cleansing creams, perfumes, baby products, pre-shave lotions and protective creams.

TRIHYDROXYSTEARIN consists of the ester of glycerine, and hydroxy stearic acid of stearic acid, used for skin conditioning purposes.

TRILAURETH-4 PHOSPHATE – derived from phosphorus compounds and is used as a surfactant and emulsifying agent.

TRIMETHYLSILOXYSILICATE – silanes, used as a skin conditioner.

TRISODIUM PHOSPHATE. This substance is used in bath salts as it ties up the calcium and magnesium ions in normal water, so making it easier for foaming and increasing the effectiveness of the surfactants present.

TRITICUM VULGARE is the EU-labelling name for a number of wheat extracts obtained from various parts of the wheat plant *Triticum vulgare*. Wheatgerm oil is one of the extracts often used in skin care products; it is the fixed oil extracted by solvents or hydraulic expression of the embryo or 'germ' of the fresh golden kernels of wheat. A good emollient, this vitamin-rich oil contains Vitamin E and lecithin, among others.

ULTRAMARINES – these are really excellent, super-fit and gorgeous looking blokes in uniform. Not really – these are synthetic colours of red, pink, blue, green and violet. For labelling purposes, the EU name for them is now **CI 77007** (hair dyes come under a different name).

UREA may be procured from human or animal urine, but in the cosmetic industry most is from synthetic sources. It is used in cosmetics as it enables other active ingredients to be absorbed more easily. It contains antiseptic, anti-inflammatory and deodorising properties. It is a natural moisturiser and found in healthy skin.

VITAMINS are organic substances essential for normal body functioning and for healthy skin and hair. A balanced supply of vitamins should be obtained by eating the correct food. The role of vitamins has come a long way since the discovery that scurvy (obvious by bleeding under the skin among other afflictions) could be prevented by consuming fruits and vegetables containing Vitamin C. They have gained a place in skin care products since it became known that Vitamin C, beta carotene and Vitamin E have antioxidant properties. It is believed that Vitamin C, beta carotene and Vitamin E can function as antioxidants when placed on the skin in a cosmetic formulation, by 'eating up' oxygen radicals which damage the dermal layer. Vitamins are added to cosmetic formulations for many reasons, some well proven, others still purported. Studies conducted on certain vitamins and their derivatives have however confirmed that they help in the battle against premature skin ageing.

VITAMIN A (**retinol**) regulates the growth and activity of epithelial cells. It increases the skin's elasticity and plays an important role in improving the texture, smoothness and firmness of the dermis and epidermis. Some cosmetic formulators say that once Vitamin A esters are in the skin they are converted to retinoic acid, which helps to reduce obvious signs of ageing.

VITAMIN B5 (**pantothenic acid**) is used in skin care products for its fast moisturising effect, healing qualities and high safety record. **Panthenol** (Vitamin B5 in its alcohol form), the active, biologically stable form of pantothenic acid, has been used in many burn creams and products for nappy rash because of its anti-inflammatory and soothing properties. Panthenol is believed to stimulate the proliferation of fibroblast cells which slows down as skin ages and also provides good moisturisation. It is used in emollients and hair conditioners.

VITAMIN C (**ascorbic acid**), when applied to the skin, can quench free radicals which can cause damage. Vitamin C helps collagen synthesis. It is also used as a preservative in certain cosmetic creams.

VITAMIN D. Deficiency of this vitamin results in rickets, a bone disease mainly of children, characterized by the softening of developing bone. It is synthesised in the skin when exposed to sunlight.

VITAMIN E LINOLEATE is a fat-soluble derivative of Vitamin E and is a superior moisturiser. It regulates the ability of the skin to resist water loss (which may decrease with advancing age) by maintaining the intercellular moisture barrier in the dermis.

VITAMIN E (**tocopherol**). High concentrations of Vitamin E occur especially in vegetable oils. Tocopherols have antioxidant properties. They are used to prevent oxidation in cosmetics, as well as in foods and pharmaceuticals. Vitamin E works as an antioxidant, protecting body cells against damage caused by free radicals. It stabilises cell membranes so is used in products designed for older skins. It also maintains the skin's connective tissue, protects the skin from UV radiation damage and nourishes it.

(Maurene writes: I don't do anything by halves, so on studying the nutritional advantages of Vitamin C, I totally overdosed. One of the two known side effects occurred – numerous tiny warts appeared along the finger nail perimeters. Not a problem under normal circumstances, however, that particular afternoon I was to demonstrate the art of cosmetic production to a small class of beauty therapists. Each student appeared enthralled and continued to watch every wart-ridden movement of my hands from close quarters. I have a strange feeling it was the warts rather than the cosmetic I was formulating that held the most fascination. The day ended with the second side effect rapidly descending upon me – I saw more of the salon loo than any other of its rooms.)

VITIS VINIFERA (grape). This is the EU-labelling name given to a number of extracts of the red grape, *Vitis vinifera*. Grape seed oil is the fixed oil obtained from crushing the seeds of the red grape. Its high linoleic content makes it suitable for use in cosmetics that nourish and moisturise. It provides emolliency in creams and lotions, and, as a fixed oil, it is used in many aromatherapy products. Grape juice is the watery substance expressed from the grape's pulp; grape leaf extract comes from the actual leaves of the vine; and grape root extract is derived from the grape plant's roots.

WATER. (See **AQUA**.)

WAXES. (See **OILS, FATS AND WAXES**.)

WITCH HAZEL. (See **HAMAMELIS VIRGINIANA**.)

XANTHAN GUM (corn starch gum) is used in cosmetic formulations as a texturiser, carrier agent and gelling agent. It is also used to stabilise and thicken cosmetic preparations. Xantham gum is produced by a pure-culture fermentation of a carbohydrate with *Xanthomonas campestris*, a bacterium found on cabbage plants.

ZEA MAYS (corn, i.e. maize) is the EU-labelling name given to a number of extracts and derivatives of corn, *Zea mays*. The oil extracted is a by-product of the grain used in milling corn. It is used in emollients. The crude oil is stable and contains tocopherols and lecithin that are good for skin conditioning. The refined oil is less stable, becoming rancid when exposed to the elements. Corn-cob meal comes from the maize cobs which are milled into powder form. An extract is derived from the kernels of *Zea mays*. There are many other extracts from this plant.

ZINC OXIDE is a white powder used most commonly in zinc and castor oil cream. It has skin-soothing and antiseptic properties, and is used as a bulking agent and colour ingredient. In its microfine form it also acts as a good sunscreen.

ZINC PHENOLSULPHONATE is a substituted phenol used in spray deodorants and pre-shave lotions for its cleansing, anti-microbial and antiseptic properties.

ZINC STEARATE. The zinc salt of stearic acid, this is a colouring additive that is white but imparts colour when in solution. It also provides anti-caking action and is a viscosity increasing agent.

ZINC SULPHATE (also known as zinc vitriol) is the result of sulphuric acid reacting with zinc. It is an inorganic salt, a cosmetic astringent and biocide that can be irritating to the skin and mucous membranes.

GLOSSARY

1-3 diol
This means that there is an oxygen/hydrogen group in the one position and an oxygen/hydrogen group in the three position within a chemical formula.

acetate
Refers to any salt or ester of acetic acid, which is the colourless, strong-smelling liquid often used in the plastic and pharmaceutical industries.

acetylated
Means that an acetate is added to the ingredient that follows, for example, acetylated lanolin.

adrenalin
The hormone that prepares the body for action.

alginates
Colloidal substances manufactured from kelp.

alkali
A hydroxide of one of the alkali metals. An aqueous solution with a pH greater than 7.

alkanolamides
Are used as stabilisers in liquid detergent formulations. They are made from the reaction of fatty amides with formaldehyde, fatty acids with hydroxy alkylamines and fatty esters with hydroxy alkylamides.

alkoxylated
A chemistry term meaning that a molecule has an alkyl (certain group of

compounds) group added via an oxygen atom.

allergen
A substance that causes an allergic reaction.

amide
A nitrogen-containing derivative of a carboxylic acid.

amines
A general class of organic compounds containing nitrogen.

amino acid
Fundamental constituent of all protein.

anaphylaxis
An abnormal reaction to a particular allergen.

anosmia
Loss of the sense of smell.

anthraquinone
A colourless crystalling quinone (a yellow solid).

anti-carcinogens
Agents that are thought to counteract substances that produce cancer.

anti-foam
An agent that cuts down or prevents foam from forming.

anti-fungal
A substance that destroys fungus.

anti-virals
Drugs that are effective against disease-causing viruses.

antioxidant
A substance that prevents a reaction with oxygen.

antiseptic
A chemical that destroys or inhibits the growth of bacteria and other micro-organisms.

aqueous
Containing water.

aromatherapy
A therapy of massaging the body utilising the aromatic properties of suitable volatile, odiferous plant extracts.

astringent
A substance that causes cells to shrink by precipitating proteins for their surfaces. Used in lotions to harden and protect the skin.

atopic
(Adjective of atopy.) Subject to an allergic reaction to certain substances.

atopy
A form of allergy in which the hypersensitivity reaction may be distant from

the region of contact with the substance (atopen) responsible. For example, a substance that is swallowed may give rise to a form of eczema, called atopic dermatitis.

autonomic nervous system
: The part of the nervous system responsible for the control of all involuntary bodily functions. (So named as this area of the body's nervous system was thought to be self-governing or spontaneous.)

autoxidation
: An oxidation reaction which proceeds only when another oxidation reaction is occurring simultaneously in the same system.

bacteria
: Simple micro-organisms.

benzaldehyde
: (See **BENZENCARBALDEHYDE**.) This is a yellowish, volatile, oily liquid which is found in almond kernels and smells of almond too. It is used in perfumery.

betaines
: These are types of surfactants first discovered in sugar beet – now they are nature identical synthetics.

biocide
: A chemical capable of killing living organisms.

carbolic acid
: A white crystalline solid. Another name for it is phenol, particularly when it is used as a disinfectant. A phenol is acidic.

carbon dioxide
: A colourless incombustible gas.

carcinogenic
: Any substance that can cause cancer.

catalyst
: A substance that speeds up a chemical reaction, without itself undergoing any permanent chemical change.

cetrimide
: A compound of ammonium used as a detergent and containing strong antiseptic properties.

cetyl   The name of a certain chemical group.

chelating agent   A chemical that binds metal ions to itself
                     and prevents them from causing product
                     deterioration. Typical use is in soaps to
                     stop copper or iron from producing blue/
                     green and red/brown specks in soap bars.
                     This is the same as a sequestering agent.

chloasma   Brown, patchy coloration of the skin.

cholesterol   A fatty acid.

coco-   Any substance derived from coconut.

cold-pressed   A method of processing oil – the oil is
                     squeezed from the plant material with
                     no added heat, ensuring a pure, high-
                     quality oil as neither heat nor solvent
                     disturbs the natural content.

colloid   A mixture of particles of one substance
                     suspended in another.

comedo   A blackhead.

comedogenic   A substance capable of inducing black-
                     heads.

compound   A substance that contains atoms of two
                     or more chemical elements, held
                     together by chemical bonds.

connective tissue   Tissue that supports, binds or separates
                     certain tissues and organs of the body.
                     Also functions as the 'packing tissue' of
                     the body.

cortisone   A steroid hormone.

DNA   Deoxyribonucleic acid – the main con-
                     stituent of the chromosomes of most
                     living organisms that controls heredity,
                     located in the cell nucleus.

demulcent   A soothing agent that calms irritation.

denaturant   A poisonous or unpleasant substance
                     added to alcoholic cosmetics to make
                     them undrinkable. It also changes
                     another substance's natural qualities or
                     characteristics.

dermatologist	Medical specialist who diagnoses and treats skin disorders.
detergents	See surfactants.
di-	Prefix meaning two.
diol	Abbreviation of dihydric alcohol (an alcohol with two hydroxyl groups).
dioxide	Any oxide that has two oxygen atoms per molecule.
eczema	A superficial inflammation of the skin, mainly affecting the epidermis.
emollient	A substance that soothes and softens the skin.
emulsifier	A surface active agent that promotes the formation of an emulsion.
emulsions	i.) Oil-in-water. When the oil or fat phase is dispersed in the water (aqueous) phase the emulsion is described as an oil-in-water system.
	ii.) Water-in-oil. When the water (aqueous) phase is dispersed in the oil phase it is described as a water-in-oil system.
endocrine	Of or denoting a gland that secretes hormones directly into the blood stream, or a hormone secreted by such a gland.
enzyme	Any of a group of complex proteins that acts as a catalyst in specific biochemical reactions.
epithelium	The tissue that covers the exterior surfaces of the body and lines hollow structures (except blood and lymphatic vessels).
essential fatty acids	A group of unsaturated acids.
ester	A compound produced by the reaction between an acid and an alcohol.
ethanol	Type of alcohol.
exfoliation	The flaking off of the outer layers of the skin.

fixed oils	These are non-volatile (unlike essential oils) vegetable and mineral oils which in their pure state do not have an odour.
flavonoid	Any of a number of naturally occurring plant pigments.
free radicals	These lead to out-of-control oxidation which damages cells.
fungicide	A substance used to destroy fungus.
gamma linoleic acid	An essential fatty acid.
genus	Category used in the classification of animals and plants.
germicide	An agent that destroys micro-organisms, particularly those causing disease.
glucose	A simple form of sugar.
glycerides	Esters of glycerol.
glycerol	A colourless, odourless syrupy liquid.
gylcoprotein	A sugar linked to a protein. These are important components of cell membranes and constituents of body fluids (e.g. mucus) that are concerned with lubrication.
histamine	A compound derived from the amino acid histidine. It is an important mediator of inflammation and is released in large amounts after skin damage.
hormones	Chemical substances produced in the endocrine system.
hydrating	To treat or impregnate with water.
hydrocarbon	A compound containing only carbon and hydrogen.
hydrogen cyanide	Also known as hydrocyanic acid or prussic acid – a colourless liquid or gas that has a characteristic smell of almonds and is extremely poisonous.
hydrogenation	The process of adding hydrogen gas to liquid oils under high pressure. It is

carried out by specialist raw material suppliers who also supply other industries, such as the cosmetics industry, where it is used to convert liquid oils to semi-solid fats at room temperature.

hydrolyzed — Means to undergo hydrolysis, which is a chemical reaction whereby a compound is split by reacting with water, aided often by acids, alkalis, heat or pressure into its components.

hydrophilic — Having an affinity with water.

hydrophobic — Repulsing water.

hydroxyl — Consisting of or containing groups of oxygen and hydrogen atoms.

hypoallergic — Little chance of reaction to an allergen.

hypothalamus — Control centre at the base of the brain responsible for autonomic functions such as hunger, thirst, body temperature, desire, etc.

intercellular cells — Situated or occurring between cells.

ions — Electrically charged atoms.

iso- — Indicating the presence of a branched chain or of another similar form.

isolates — Substances in uncombined form.

keratinocytes — Cells filled with keratin, the fibrous protein which forms the body's horny tissues.

keratinization — The process by which the cells become horny due to their deposition of keratin within them.

kernel — This is a hard seed which is of food value to humans and animals.

lecithin — A group of substances present in many plants and animal tissues.

limbic system — Complex system in the brain concerned with emotion, hunger and sex.

linoleic acid — One of the omega-6 family of essential fatty acids.

linolenic acid	Another essential fatty acid – part of the omega-3 family.
lipids	General term to describe any of a group of organic compounds that are esters of fatty acids or similar substances.
lipoproteins	Particles made of proteins and lipids which enable insoluble fats to be transported in the blood stream.
malic acid	A substance found in many fruits.
mast cells	Large cells in the connective tissue with coarse, cytoplasmic granules. These could contain the chemicals herapin, histamine and seretonin, which are released during an allergic response.
melanocyte	A cell within the epidermis of the skin which produces the dark-brown pigment melanin.
micronutrients	Vitamins and minerals together are called this.
moisturiser	Holds in or retains the moisture in the skin.
monopolysaccharide	A complex of proteins.
monosaccharide	A simple sugar.
monounsaturated	Of a group of vegetable oils such as olive oil which have a neutral effect on cholesterol in the body.
neutralise	To make chemically or electrically neutral.
nitrates	Chemical compounds containing nitrogen.
non-comedogenic	Does not produce comedones (blackheads).
non-sensitizing	Does not render a person sensitive to foreign substances.
olfactory	Of or relating to the sense of smell.
opacifying	To use a substance which renders a liquid impervious to light rays.

organic   Produced by or found in plants or animals. In chemistry, belonging to a class of chemical compounds which are formed from carbon.

oxy-   Prefix meaning an oxygen bridge is present.

phenol   A white crystalline derivative of benzene, an aromatic compound. Belongs to a class of chemical compounds which are formed from carbon, as are all organic chemicals.

pheromone   A chemical substance secreted externally by certain animals which elicit a specific response from others of the same species.

phospholipids   A major component of cell membranes. They have a water-attracting and fat-attracting ability. They are lipids containing a phosphate group as part of the molecule.

poly-   Prefix meaning many.

polymers   Naturally occurring substances such as rubber, starch found in plants, and glycogen found in animals, or synthetic compounds such as Perspex, which are formed by chemical reactions – many molecules of the same kind are joined together.

polysaccharide   A carbohydrate formed from many monosaccharides joined together in long linear or branched chains.

polyunsaturated fat   Form of fat found in high levels in corn oil, sunflower oil and in nuts and oily fish – contains carbon chains with many carbon to carbon double bonds.

precursor   A chemical substance that is used to assemble another more important substance.

prostaglandins — Compounds found in mammalian organs, tissues and secretions and in some simple animals like the soft coral. They are involved in the long-term inflammatory response in damaged tissue. They have a number of different physiological effects including promoting fever and pain and affect the immune system.

pro-vitamin — A substance which is not itself a vitamin but can be converted to a vitamin in the body.

quaternary ammonium compound — A surfactant with bactericidal action.

saponified — A chemical reaction in which a fat is converted into a soap by treatment with alkali.

saturated — Relates to compounds containing double or triple bonds that do not easily undergo additional reactions.

sebum — The oily substance secreted by the sebaceous glands.

sequestering agent — A preservative that prevents physical or chemical changes affecting a product's colour, appearance, flavour or texture. This is the same as a chelating agent.

silane — Also called silicane – a colourless gas which is insoluble in water.

skin conditioning agent — An ingredient of cream or lotion that softens the skin.

solubilizer — Emulsifier.

solute — The substance dissolved in a solution.

solvent — In a solution, the substance which dissolves the solute and usually makes up the bulk of the solution.

squames — Scales from the hard layer of the epidermis (i.e. dead skin).

styptic — A substance used to stop bleeding.

subcutaneous — Beneath the skin.

substituted — Means that an element or group has been replaced by another in a chemical structure.

sulphates — Any compound containing an ionic oxy-sulphur species.

surfactants — Surface active agents – these have, owing to the water-liking and oil-liking parts in their molecules, the ability to 'allow' water and oil materials to mix (emulsify). They reduce the surface tension of a liquid, so allowing it to foam or penetrate solids. Some are used in household cleaning materials, some are designed to dissolve in oil and grease, and some are designed to reduce static in fabric softeners. In cosmetics they are used in shampoos and lotions.

synthetic — Made initially by chemical reaction.

tartrate — A salt or ester of tartaric acid, which is a crystalline, naturally occurring carboxylic acid. It can be obtained from the tartar deposits of wine vats, and is also used in baking powders and is added to various foods.

terpenes — These are all naturally occurring hydrocarbons derived from plants. These compounds are known as monoterpenes, sesquiterpenes, diterpines, etc. depending on the chemical arrangements.

tocopherol — Substance that has vitamin activity and can protect unsaturated lipids against oxidisation.

topical — Local. Used for the route of administration of a drug that is applied directly to the parts being treated.

tri-   Prefix meaning three.

unsaponifiables   Most natural fats are present in their
                    raw form as triglycerides (i.e. a glycerol
                    molecule with ester groupings on each
                    hydroxyl group). When a triglyceride is
                    reacted with sodium hydroxide during
                    soap-making, it breaks down to glycerol
                    and the corresponding fatty acids. How-
                    ever, natural fats often contain materials
                    which do not break down when acted
                    upon by sodium hydroxide. When iso-
                    lated at the end of soap-making, these
                    materials are called the unsaponifiable
                    fraction and, hence, unsaponifiables.

urticaria   A skin condition which appears as
                    itchy, red or whitish raised patches and
                    is usually caused by an allergy. It is also
                    known as hives or nettle rash.

vasoconstrictor   An agent which causes narrowing of the
                    blood vessels and therefore a decrease
                    in blood flow.

viscosity   The state of being viscous.

viscous   Of liquids – thick and sticky.

INDEX

Items explained in Chapter 8 are not indexed here.

A

Acetate, 175
Acetylated, 175
Acne, 38
Adrenalin, 175
Aftershave lotions, 56–57
Alginates, 175
Alkali, 175
Alkanolamides, 175
Alkoxylated, 175–176
Allergen, 176
Allergic reactions, 81–84
Amide, 176
Amines, 176
Amino acid, 176
Anaphylaxis, 176
Animal ingredients, 78, 79–80, 88–89
Anosmia, 176
Anthraquinone, 176
Anti-ageing, 48
Anti-carcinogens, 176
Anti-foam, 176
Anti-fungal, 176
Anti-virals, 176
Anti-wrinkle cream, 48
Antioxidant, 176
Antiperspirants, 53, 54
Antiseptic, 176
Aqueous, 176
Aromatherapy, 69

Astringents, 44, 45, 176
Atopic, 176
Atopy, 176–177
Autonomic nervous system, 177
Autoxidation, 177

B

Baby products, 57
Bacteria, 32, 177
Barrier preparations, 49
Bath products, 57–61
Benzaldehyde, 177
Betaines, 177
Biocide, 177
Burns, 36–37

C

Cancer, 38, 61
Carbolic acid, 177
Carbon dioxide, 177
Carcinogenic, 177
Catalyst, 177
Cetrimide, 177
Cetyl, 178
Chelating agent, 178
Chloasma, 178
Cholesterol, 178
Cleansing, 41–44
    cream, 43
    lotion, 42–43
    milk, 42–43

Coco-, 178
Cold cream, 18, 43
Cold-pressed, 178
Collagen injections, 48
Colloid, 178
Combination skin, 29
Comedo, 178
Compound, 178
Connective tissue, 178
Contamination, 83–84
Cortisone, 178

D
DNA, 178
Demulcent, 178
Denaturant, 178
Deodorant, 52–54
   bar, 42
Dermatologist, 179
Dermis, 23–24
Detergents, 179
Di-, 179
Diol, 179
   , 1–3, 175
Dioxide, 179
Dry skin, 29, 47, 48

E
Eczema, 30, 179
Emollient, 179
Emulsifier, 179
Emulsions, 179
Endocrine, 179
Enzyme, 179
Epidermis, 23
Epithelium, 179
Essential fatty acids, 179
Ester, 179
Exfoliants, 43–44
Exfoliation, 179
Eye creams, 48–49
   make-up remover, 44

F
Facial scrub, 43
   wash, foaming, 42
Fixative, 89
Fixed oils, 180

Flavonoid, 180
Foot products, 50–52
Foundation cream, 49
FRAME, 71
Free radicals, 37–38, 180
Fresheners, 44
Fungicide, 180

G
Gamma linoleic acid, 180
Genus, 180
Germicide, 180
Glucose, 180
Glycerides, 180
Glycerine, 40
Glycerol, 180
Glycoprotein, 180

H
Hand creams, 49–50
Histamine, 180
Hormones, 180
Hydrating, 180
Hydrocarbon, 180
Hydrogen cyanide, 180
Hydrogenation, 180–181
Hydrolyzed, 181
Hydrophilic, 181
Hydrophobic, 181
Hydroxyl, 181
Hypoallergic, 181
Hypothalamus, 181

I
INCI, 69
Intercellular cells, 181
Irritation, 81–82
Iso-, 181
Isolates, 181

K
Keratinocytes, 181
Keratinization, 181
Kernel, 181

L
Lecithin, 181
Legislation, 68 *et seq.*

Lice, 32
Limbic system, 181
Linoleic acid, 181
Linolenic acid, 182
Lipid-free cleansers, 42
Lipids, 39, 182
Lipoproteins, 182
Liposomes, 46
Liquid soaps, 42

M

Malic acid, 182
Masques, 64–66
Massage, 67
Mast cells, 182
Medicines, 68
Melanocyte, 182
Micronutrients, 182
Mites, 30–32
Moisturisers, 45–49, 182
Monopolysaccharide, 182
Monosaccharide, 182
Monounsaturated, 182

N

Natural ingredients, 78–79
    moisturising factor, 25–26
Nature identical ingredients, 78
Neutralise, 182
Nitrates, 182
Non-comedogenic, 182
Non-sensitizing, 182
Normal skin, 29, 47

O

Oily skin, 29, 47
Olfactory, 182
Opacifying, 182
Organic, 183
Oxy-, 182

P

Perfume, 85–90
pH balance, 27–28
Phenol, 183
Pheromone, 183
Phospholipids, 183
Pollution, 36

Poly-, 183
Polymers, 183
Polysaccharide, 183
Polyunsaturated fat, 183
Precursor, 183
Pro-vitamin, 184
Prostaglandins, 184

Q

Quaternary ammonium compound,
    184

S

Saponified, 184
Saturated, 184
Sebum, 184
Sensitization, 83
Sequestering agent, 184
Serums, 47–48
Shaving products, 54–57
Silane, 184
Skin conditioning agent, 184
    fresheners, 45
Smoking, 36
Soap, 41
    , liquid, 42
    , soapless, 41
Solubilizer, 184
Solute, 184
Solvent, 184
Squames, 184
Styptic, 185
Subcutaneous, 185
Substituted, 185
Sulphates, 185
Sun, 34–36
    care products, 61–64
Surfactants, 185
Syndet bar, 42
Synthetic, 185
    ingredients, 78
Systemic allergic reaction, 82–83

T

Tartrate, 185
Terpenes, 185
Tocopherol, 185
Toners, 44–45

Tonics, 45
Topical, 185–186
Tri-, 186

U
Ultra violet rays, 34–36, 61–62
Unsaponifiables, 186
Urticaria, 186

V
Vanishing cream, 49
Vasoconstrictor, 186

Viruses, 33
Viscosity, 186
Viscous, 186

W
Warts, 33
Wrinkles, 34–35, 48

Y
Yeast, 32–33

In the same series

STOP BINGEING!
Stay in control of your eating
by Lee Janogly

Are you a binge eater?

Have you ever said, "I'll start again tomorrow"? If so, ordinary diet books do not work for you; just when your latest diet seems to be succeeding, you blow it all with a massive binge, cramming in every fattening food you can lay your hands on!

If you recognise this destructive cycle of dieting – craving – bingeing – guilt – anger – misery, then *this book will set you free*; allowing you to take control of your life, rather than letting your life be controlled by food. A simple, six point plan enables *you* to choose *what* you eat, *when* and *how much*, whilst case studies reveal just how others in your situation have *beaten the binge for good*.

"... a compelling air of authenticity ... no recipes and no 'nutri-babble', just a sensitive and sensible blueprint ... that could free you for good of the misery of binge eating."

Sunday Times Style Magazine

Uniform with this book

RIGHT WAY
PUBLISHING POLICY

HOW WE SELECT TITLES

RIGHT WAY consider carefully every deserving manuscript. Where an author is an authority on his subject but an inexperienced writer, we provide first-class editorial help. The standards we set make sure that every **RIGHT WAY** book is practical, easy to understand, concise, informative and delightful to read. Our specialist artists are skilled at creating simple illustrations which augment the text wherever necessary.

CONSISTENT QUALITY

At every reprint our books are updated where appropriate, giving our authors the opportunity to include new information.

FAST DELIVERY

We sell **RIGHT WAY** books to the best bookshops throughout the world. It may be that your bookseller has run out of stock of a particular title. If so, he can order more from us at any time – we have a fine reputation for ''same day'' despatch, and we supply any order, however small (even a single copy), to any bookseller who has an account with us. We prefer you to buy from your bookseller, as this reminds him of the strong underlying public demand for **RIGHT WAY** books. However, you can order direct from us by post or by phone with a credit card.

FREE

If you would like an up-to-date list of all **RIGHT WAY** titles currently available, please send a stamped self-addressed envelope to ELLIOT RIGHT WAY BOOKS, BRIGHTON ROAD, LOWER KINGSWOOD, TADWORTH, SURREY, KT20 6TD, U.K.
or visit our web site at www.right-way.co.uk